MW01094595

Are You Useful?

*A Freethinker's Guide to Creating
a Philosophy of Strength*

Chip Conrad

Mental Meat Heads Publications
Birmingham/Sacramento

This book is self-published. This means we can skip all the formal stuff here, like listing the title again. You've seen it at least twice so far, if you've been paying attention.

ISBN: 978-1-365-32380-5
First printing August 2016
Copyright 2016 Chip Conrad

BodyTribe/Mental Meat Heads Publications
1106 North D Street, #7
Sacramento, CA 95811 USA

At some point this book will be a dog-eared, highlighted pulp bulge in your backpack that you will take with you everywhere as a guidebook to life (or the electronic equivalent of that). As if Catcher in the Rye, Howl, and your favorite Krishnamurti book were all rolled up into one complete, hubris-free package of wisdom, rebellion, and reference. To assist this responsibility, I've included a handy list of chapters on the next page, sometimes known as a table of contents. Sure, eventually you'll have this memorized, at which point you could use this page for scribbling important notes and thoughts and schemes.

Table of Contents

Intro

I love a good intro. Perhaps I'm in the minority, but the intro of a book is often my favorite part, second maybe to footnotes (which you'll soon discover). The intro is intimate, as if the author and the reader are enjoying a spot of tea together before the actual reading commences. This is a time for sharing, for bonding, and the quickest glimpse into the personality of the weirdo who covered these pages with words and ideas. It may behoove me, said weirdo in this case, to shut up about the intro, especially with this confession. I'm about to squeeze in some significant information that, although paramount to the premise of this book, was almost left out. Forgotten. It took a concentrated perusing of a very late draft to realize my mistake. I'm now sneaking it into the intro as an attempt to play it off. Let's pretend it was supposed to be here the entire time. Just chatting, you and me. Some honey for your tea, perhaps?

This new mission puts a fair amount of pressure on the intro to establish some meaty foundation for the rest of what follows. What that says about me I have no idea, but I hope you're with me so far. Here's hoping whoever ends up writing the foreword to this has done a darn fine job of entertaining you up until this point. The foreword: An author's opening act.

Oh. No foreward? Ok, intro... the pressure's on.

The main act now begins with a philosophical doozy explained through the brain of a slow but determined physical culturist who will most undoubtedly frustrate Aristotelian scholars into dialectic spasms. It begins with my interpretation (some would call it bastardization) of a $2 word.

In his book **Contemporary Athletics and Ancient Greek Ideals**, Daniel A. Dombrowski waxes professorly about the Greek word *hylomorphism*, which seems to have a definition along the lines of the higher-self and the lower-self completing each other. Some would say it could mean the physical and metaphysical in an eternal collective, an ideal symbiosis that requires us to let the mind, body, and spirit have a bit more communication between each other than just weekend visits and holiday parties.

If mind/body/spirit reeks a little of self-help, new age-y, naked-dancing-in-the-patchouli circle (like that's a bad thing), then maybe cognitive/physical/emotional would have a more antiseptic, clinical shine to it that connects you to terra firma a bit better. Same thing, different language.

One way we can all relate to how our humanness is a co-op rather than a Cartesian thought game would be to ponder the phrase "stressed-out." Is that a mind, body, or spirit phenomenon? I'm sure you nailed it. D) All of the above. You can watch the hylomorphic self in action, although usually spiraling into disunity, through being stressed-out, as the whole unravels into its various parts. Stressed-out is an example of how everything is affected, and interacts accordingly, albeit not in a copacetic, appealing way. Now how do we find the inverse of that? I'm going to make the case that our movement and strength journey is a major player in our complete "all-at-once" humanness game, what we often refer to as the Holistic Athlete, although movement ambassador Gregory Dorado uses the term Authentic Body, which I will probably steal and use synonymously throughout this book[1].

Joy through embodiment. Strength as tribal. Becoming rather than just existing. Did I lose some of you? I hope not.

Dombrowski offers a little wordplay that a young Wittgenstein might've found playfully insightful. It's an

---

[1] I'll make a case for "holistic" being a good word choice in its pure, unmarketed form, but there is a sheen of cliché to it that makes me like the term "authentic" as a viable replacement.

intellectually tricky comparison, finding the difference between what makes an athlete virtuous versus making an athletic life virtuous. In the second version, athletics are taken too seriously, believing that the physical will be all there is. In the first version, the true athlete understands that his or her *askeseis* (groovy term for physical training) isn't complete without *theorousa*, your Jeopardy word for contemplation. Our gym culture today is perpetuating the 'athletic life.' Living for the gym/sport/activity. As opposed to being an athlete, which, through hylomorphic eyes, means using the gym/sport/activity to actually live.

The difference, which at first seems subtle, is life changing.

How Netflix Changed my Life

What would you say if you had 18 minutes to pitch whatever you wanted to 1000+ people who leaked money and had resources to possibly make your biggest dreams come true? About a decade ago, Netflix produced a documentary introducing most of the world to the now familiar TED talks. These days this famous collection of speeches is ubiquitous social media gold. But 10 years ago, most of us were still unaware of the power of this potent collection of mini-lectures.

The documentary explained how the Talks offered the 18-minute possibility to folks far smarter than I to pitch a cause, idea, or dream that had earth-changing consequences to some seriously rich folks who could fund the transformation. Netflix plopped the DVD in my mailbox[2], somehow usurping season 1 of The Sopranos, and I was blown away. Not only were the presentations spellbinding, but the fact that a roomful of folks, whose wealth and power could collectively rival our GNP, were there to have a positive influence on our planet restored some drooping faith in humanity.

---

[2] These were the pre-streaming days of Netflix, after all.

TED is pretty green. Not wet-behind-the-ears, but *green*. TED is a dialog for planetary sustainability, along with some cool new toys that stroke the inner geek in many of us and make the shindig a little more fun. Each presenter has 18 minutes to pitch an idea, gadget or plan to possibly change the world, and the attendees have the resources and money (and, *hallelujah*, the desire) to get the party started.

Upon learning about the TED Talks, I began dreaming a little bit, just as I bet you would've.

Let's say a room full of 1000 rich, smart, and powerful people could be gathered with the sole intent of supporting positive change (by which my jaded little heart was pleasantly surprised). Let's say these folks were interested in intelligent ideas of possibility that could have effect on the sustainability of the planet, and they could bankroll almost any mountain that needed moving or any dream that sounded plausible.

Let's say I'm standing in front of them.

Go...

What Would the Message Be?

Few things in life are as humbling as questioning the value of your mission. My little revolution against the commercial fitness industry is a very first-world luxury. With food in my belly (barely) and a roof over my head (for now) I can safely charge into the fray of mainstream consumerism and hubris with sword (or dumbbell) in hand, ready to slay the corporate dragons.

So what? **Am I** trying to raise the level of my silly little profession from a service industry to philosophical physiology, like a quest for realization through physical empowerment? Thanks to this TED Talks fantasy, I was questioning if this was a pretty weak brand of activism.

Thankfully, my journey isn't a new one, and there are some footsteps to follow:

"Mind and body should be viewed as the two well-fitting halves of a perfect whole, designed and planned in perfect harmony, mutually to sustain and support each other, and equally worth of our unwearied care and attention in perfecting." - Julia Thomas, 1892

We can find cases where societies throughout history embraced the importance of promoting physical well being as a basic tenet of life. For every culture that is struggling for basic needs, another is frittering away theirs, diving headlong into an oblivion reserved for classic squanderers like Nero and Caligula. Perhaps my little role within our tribe is to offer important alternatives to taking our physical beings for granted and promoting the concept that, sans the politics of primping, an increased physical awareness can lead to higher forms of thought and creativity. One case we'll make is that there is no reason NOT to be strong.

So, yes. there is a need to be concerned for our own society's physical abilities, our own tribe's connection and relationship between minds and bodies, and a realization that our lessons might be different from other tribes, but not less important. Granted, this may be me simply justifying my own tiny quest here, but a boy's still gotta dream, right?

To begin our journey, let's examine a common assumption in the workout world, which lacks some bulk in its premise. It's an assumption with so much volume and repetition behind it that it's often spoken as absolute fact:

A good workout = a better life.

This assumption, unfortunately, might be horse pucky. At least there is far less evidence to support this premise than one might think. If the marketing arm of the Fitness Industrial Complex is to be believed, your gym membership may as well be a free pass to Awesome Camp, where masters of the universe are forged daily. The case we'll make in this book, though, is that the entire industry needs a major makeover to guarantee any sort of true transformation.

I know, I know…. Ya just wanna get your lift on and feel good about yourself for a job well done. I get it. All this babblygunk about mind and body should be dealt with by lab coats or on therapy couches. Meanwhile, let's get our WOD time down or our max squat up and walk away a little bit better. As you'll discover, the intensity of any rendezvous with your strength toy box creates a key opportunity to tap into yourself far beyond the limp handshake or frail head nod our minds and bodies usually give each other. The problem is we often skip that chance to embrace the dialog or nurture a strong relationship.

Sure, a good workout will make you feel pretty groovy. That seems to be fairly consistent. But accomplishments in the gym and personal empowerment through movement aren't quite synonymous. I've been accused of asking too much in this regard, but I'm surprised how many people aren't asking enough. Why not pursue the process and get even more out of it?

That is only step one. Does physical strength contribute to metaphysical completeness? Comparing notes between science and anecdote, there seems to be a big consensus towards 'maybe?' Then what?

After preaching about personal empowerment through movement for quite some time, thinking about being on the TED stage really stabbed that question right into my thinky feely bits. But. Then. What?

A question began a much bigger journey for me: Does personal empowerment even exist without somehow benefitting the tribe?

The answer was exciting and humbling: No.

Boom. In one quick realization it was back to being a philosophical neophyte for this strength geek. I was returning to kindergarten, and right after writing my first book. It's like I graduated to being a beginner.

Chances are if you're reading these words, you've already strapped on your boots and triple checked the maps for this adventure. Maybe you already like strength and plan on acquiring more. If you're reading this, strength and ability might no longer hide their secrets from you and perhaps you understand many of the lessons and benefits to be had. What steps will it take to guarantee a benefit for your tribe as well? That's my current line of questioning.

We're discussing and defining purpose, tribe, and intensity, among other things. The steps are in place to realize that our training has a far greater purpose beyond our gym and ourselves. And the current industry needs to be left far behind.

1. Dissent Against The Industrial Complex

In the almost 10 years since I wrote my first book, the philosophy of BodyTribe, my movement sanctuary where the thoughts are sublime and the actions are bold, made a small but very important step. Outward. We moved from being a fringe player in the game we call the Fitness Industrial Complex to deciding to live outside the industry, renouncing its foundations and existing as an individual entity of thought and movement that wanted to see the industry's demise... or at least we hoped for it to change.

Frankly, we stepped aside, turned around, and politely screamed "YOU'RE DOING IT ALL WRONG!"

In a review of artist Laurie Anderson, performance art as a whole was described as an ideal of 'taking the art out of the institution.' I'd like to do that with fitness and movement - give it room to breathe, for better or for worse, and let labels and categories grow organically, if they have to exist at all.

My first book now has a smell of yesterday to it. I took some chunks that were foundational to the continuing growth of our philosophy at BodyTribe and remixed them, fleshing them out with a nice sauté of new thought and action (and thyme. Everything's better with thyme).

Welcome. I mean that. Welcome, everyone. Whether you've been steeped in the FIC for years, or a fringe member keeping an eye on the backdoor, or maybe a long time listener/first time caller, perhaps finally deciding to reacquaint yourself with your body after a timeline of poorer choices you're a tad embarrassed about. Awesome. This book may have the mission of unhinging the dogmas of current ambassadors of the strength and movement world, but the non-participatory sections of our population might find a worthy nugget or two in these pages as well.

Welcome! You're all our kind of peeps. Let's chat.

The 7 REAL Biggest Mistakes

Clickbait. Sounds almost naughty, but you'll recognize it as part of our modern lexicon, meaning the technique of loading an online article title for our 3-second attention spans to be tempted, and often suckered, into making said article a priority for our eyes and brains (and usually potential advertising dollars). We're bombarded with the things we MUST do and the things we MUST NEVER do, and if this list of absolutes has any relation to our passion, then we will clicky-clicky with abandon, and pray that our current journey is validated by what this summarizing list of dogma will tell us.

In a recent incarnation of this tactic, those of us who have a hankering for movement and strength might find ourselves wanting to open something discussing the clickybaity concept of the BIGGEST MISTAKES!! The things you should NEVER DO! Because, I dunno... locusts? Plague? Bad stuff happens when you DO THESE THINGS! So DON'T. It would behoove you to click here to find out what they are!!

These online seductions are floating all around the interwebs loosely veiled as discussions amongst the coaches of our modern fitness industrial protocols about doing what they do better. Sounds good, right? As soon as we believe our shit don't stink, then we're neck deep in ego poop. Journey over. Perhaps a little self-assessment is a darn fine thing.

Help, apparently, is here, since these clickbait saviors would call out those monstrous mistakes, the ones that are akin to leaving your puppy in a hot car or letting your child play on the freeway. Disastrous mistakes that are just short of accidentally summoning Cthulhu. Giant faux pas in technique, program design, and motivation that us trainers and gym members should consider fixing. Or else!

If a program comes from an authentic philosophical foundation, then these particular mistakes wouldn't have any merit for a hyperbolic blog title. Heck, they wouldn't exist at all.

Of course, here's my list below. I know... you're still wondering what the heck a 'authentic philosophical foundation' is in regards to your fitness program. Don't worry. We'll get there. But first (if this were a website) click here, or you'll be eaten by a walrus!

The 7 Biggest Mistakes Ever in the Universe for Fitness Folks!

The real mistakes are not exclusive to any particular fitness culture. The trends of fitness, from the common pop-fitness to the growing alt-fitness world, have reached far and wide, and we're going to make a case for trashing it all and starting over. One of the paths to joy is to avoid the trappings of any institution, and the Fitness Industrial Complex is on that list.

Does this include you? Well it includes me. I write as a reminder to myself first and foremost. Maybe you've transcended the examples given. Good for you, enlightened one. Meanwhile, I, personally, still have work to do.

This ridiculous list is simply a summary of what we're going to be covering in this book. Our true mistakes would be major flaws in the foundations of our conviction, weaknesses in thought, and the poor conceptualized programming that results from the philosophy itself, or lack thereof. As we'll reiterate throughout this treatise, the *Why* beats all. Of course, that leads us to mistake #1...

1) Having no purpose. At least not completely defining our purpose. The Why is often forgotten in the quest for What and How. Yet without the Why, the What and How serve as much purpose as governmental red tape or bad pop music. Stuff that keeps us busy as a distraction from what we really need.

We're going to make a case that life is out there somewhere, so let's train for it. The caveat being that if we haven't a system that creates the direct correlation between life and our movement practice, it will only happen by happy accident, if at all. Despite the premise used as marketing hype we discussed in the riveting intro (A good workout = a better life), there is little evidence that supports a strong correlation between how we workout and how we live, no matter how functional a program might seem on paper.

How do we train to live, as opposed to living to train?

Our definitions of strength and fitness need to be far greater than what is on the homepage of a system's website, or in textbooks, or taught in trainer certification courses. In fact they need to be personal, carved from the nitty gritty experience of our time on this big blue party fun ball, and crafted from getting our calloused hands dirty and our curious minds exploded. If we have no concept of the physical influencing and bettering the metaphysical, then we're just trendy fitness hamsters on a wheel (or under a barbell).

2) Believing that exhaustion is the desired outcome.
Doing more before doing better is simply poor training. Knowing the difference between a hard workout and a good workout is the difference between wasting your time being busy versus actually being productive and life affirming. A good workout will be hard, but not all hard workouts are good.

Empowerment is, indeed, a study in intensity... something we'll talk quite a bit about.

3) Thinking you know more than you do. A big example of this is how liberally the term 'coach' is being tossed around these days. Ya gotta earn that one. Sorry kid, but a couple years of working out, a weekend certification, and a shiny new blog or YouTube channel gives no one the right to be a "coach." This term used to be the athletic version of Sensei, something earned after years of apprenticeship, study, and being constantly ass-deep in the practice and perpetuation of the art. When did it turn into kids thinking they had the chops to teach (or, in many cases, not so much 'teach' as 'monitor') complicated movement patterns done for speed by large groups of people?

4) Having no foundation program. We all need a system of checks and balances for our training to be an ongoing journey of mastery. Covet the basics, both physical and metaphysical, and let it take you a lifetime.

5) Having no program, period. Having a plan from point A to point B, C and Z... that's programming. Randomly throwing ideas together isn't. Random training produces random results. Sure, be malleable, but have a plan.

6) Believing what you're doing is all there is. Not only has your practice been done before, but often better. Plus, there are more movements and techniques than our tiny brains can hold onto. Let yourself engage in new movement challenges often. This, of course, doesn't mean just adding more superfluous reps to the drudgery you're currently comfortable with. Move. In many ways. For many reasons. Your body wants to move in millions of ways, more than your brain can even come up with. Are you stuck doing the same patterns all the time?

This exploration, of course, means also addressing your motivations and ambitions. Dream a little! See the planet as your playground of embodiment, and explore the crap out of it through movement and participation. Your lessons are limited if your movements are. Your dreams are stuck if your experiences don't expand more.

Halfway around the planet from my little hovel here in California, movement practitioner Rannoch Donald has this to say:

> "Interesting how an affectation of movement or thought can spread through a group of people. Idiosyncratic, egocentric ideas and forms are so quickly adopted with so little consideration that confirmation is often just bias in disguise.
>
> [Let's ask] Does this reflect my experience? Does this reflect my current knowledge?
>
> Adopt and adapt, but don't forget abandon! That is where your wildness lives.
>
> The eagerness to belong should not cloud our potential to be authentic."

7) Not having Tribe in mind. Since personal empowerment doesn't exist without somehow bettering the tribe, we need to continue asking the question: am I useful?

2. The Reasons We Move

The chapter somewhere further on in this pastiche called Routine versus Ritual has always been the mission statement of BodyTribe, the introduction towards our particular brand of fitness comedy. It was the first chapter of the original book, although here it makes sense a little later on. See? Evolution.

What led me to those realizations that inspired that chapter, asks the curious reader? Here is the first draft preface, or in modern terms, the `prequel,' to how BodyTribe started...

So many good stories begin on a mountain or under a tree, so far be it for me to be the exception. There is a mountain ridge amongst the Sierra range that is modest in size and user friendly. It is an intermediate hike to the crest which provides a nifty view of Serene Lakes on one side and Lake Norden on the other, not to mention the numerous other mountains, valleys and acres of trees that can be seen for miles in all directions. This ridge probably has a name, but I knew it simply as a mountain that rose up between a ring of cross country ski trails that circled its base during the winter. If, for the sake of organization, you'd like a name for it, let's call it Sherry.

I was about 10 kilometers from the resort's lodge, deep in the woods and at the far end of Sherry one day when I decided that, since it was there, I might as well climb it/her. It was early spring. This meant the snow was solid ice in the morning and slush by late afternoon. In the ice stage, it was easy to ski off trail, if you had a modicum of familiarity with the `skating' style of cross country skiing. I did, so up the mountain

I went, skating the snow/ice, eventually reaching the top of the ridge.

Once the climb was made, the rolling peaks of Sherry's top were a pleasure to ski, and the view had few equals, at points a 360 panorama of one of the finest, most piquant mountain ranges in the world. I rested on a giant rock, not knowing that it would be the location for an epiphany that would lock me there for several hours.

Sherry had many things to teach me.

To Nature, Humans are not beautiful creatures. We're fond of ourselves, and sometimes each other, but the rest of the planet, the non-human majority, doesn't view us as such. Naked, we're not built to tolerate most climates. We offer no real place on any food chain. We're not essential to any original ecology (in fact we tend to destroy any environment we inhabit). Also, when compared to other species in the grand scheme, we aren't really that great to look at.

Why are we still around? For reasons beyond our understanding, we possess a cognitive gift more developed (arguably) than anything else on the planet. The theories explaining our `how' have been debated since we first realized we could communicate beyond grunts. More exciting, though, is figuring out the `Why.'

Sitting on that rock overlooking vast sections of organic pulchritude drove me to think a little. Admitting our inherent ugliness and lack of importance to an otherwise thriving and autonomous planet was a tough step. We all want to feel needed, but having the bosom of the Earth Mother staring at me from all angles imparted a strong message that if we didn't exist on the planet, her survival would actually be easier.

We, probably sensing our worthlessness in some corner of our unconsciousness, have made dangerous decisions about how to assert ourselves. We've decided as a species to *claim* worth through domination, the classic sign of the insecure bully. The irony is lost on us that our punk-ass attempts at commanding the planet eventually show us how dependent we are *on* the planet. At that point our seemingly infinite capacity for logic and rationalization have degenerated into greed, and we're too power-drunk to admit to our natural, birth given ugliness.

The Hollywood scenario would look like this: the battered, bloodied hero, while spitting out a broken tooth and trying to get up off the ground, starts to laugh. The villain, feeling inches from victory, stops the pummeling for a minute to ask where the humor is in the present situation, just as he gets splattered by a train that the hero saw approaching the whole time.

Right now we can hear the planet giggling under our clenched fists.

Even the lifetime ago (when I was still in my 20's) when I was on top of Sherry, nature was laughing at us, and had been for some time. My solitary perch upon her peaks gave me some unexpected insight as to what might really be our purpose as a species. I was surrounded by nature's beautiful determination, as everything within visual distance had a place in the glory I was witnessing. In other words, where I was wouldn't be what it was without everything I could see at that point, from the diminutive, almost invisible spiders that wanted me to get the hell off their rock to the massive range of peaks on the other side of the valley daring me to climb on them. The only one not serving a purpose would be this pale, stinky ape sitting on the rock with giant sticks on his feet and obnoxious colored boots.

Understanding that there was beauty in the usefulness and cohesiveness of everything became simple. It all had purpose. Except for me.

Stop me if you've heard something similar: If a tree lived in a forest and no one was around to see it, would it really exist?

Oxygen might have been a little sparse up there at 8,000 feet, making the spam and lime jello globe vibrating between my ears a little more privy to wackiness, but it wasn't hard to believe that Sherry was telling me something. Perhaps this realization reeked of cliché, but I was being schooled by nature. The lesson seemed to be that too many of our philosophical pursuits are as selfish as our quests for planet domination. In other words, yes, that tree exists, whether it falls and we don't hear it or it stands for several hundred years hanging out with peers, and no human eye ever beholds it.

Cogito ergo so what?

What good are we then? If we don't have an instant place in the order of nature, then let's look at the tools we were given, this ability to create thought, and see how it might be better used.

First, let's define beauty as it relates to our scenario here. Beyond human aesthetic perception, let's define it also as being an integral part in nature. This definition explains how, to the planet, we're ugly and a dung beetle is, in its own way, hot. Beauty, to this big blue ball, is the utilitarian synergy of living things. With a little squinting, we can probably see that too.

Guess what we can do? Better, in fact that probably any other creature on earth? We can *create* beauty, in both the aesthetic perception sense, through art and ideas, and in our relationships, to each other and the planet. Unlike the rest of the planet which has birth-given usefulness, our magic seems to be that we can dream and build what is useful, maybe even integral, to the interpersonal systems we're part of. We've been given this ability, this quest, and the cognitive understanding to realize it. We're more verb than noun, more process than object. How do we make that beautiful?

Let's embrace this groovy mission Again, how we got this power isn't really the big question. Whatever deity or beaker-and-slide-ruler you want to put stock in doesn't change the fact that our real challenge is how we use this gift.

Lawrence Krauss will be the first to tell you that chances are we came from nothing and there is an even gooder chance we're completely insignificant to the big picture. Yet his reaction to this is to celebrate. This privilege we have to BE, this brain we're given to believe what we need to believe to get through our ridiculously limited time on this dance party Earth, this honor of having a potentially glorious organic machine to get our amazing brains and their perpetual thoughts from point A to point B, and have a blast doing it – this should all be cause for celebration. THAT'S what creating beauty for a human is... being active in our joy for what we *do* have.

This idea of celebrating our truncated timeline is the difference between just existing and truly Being. We're surrounded by a constant parade of existence, with lots of energy, hype, and stimuli achieving nothing at all. We're masters of creating so much unnecessary work that we're under the false impression that we're productive

Truth is, we're just busy.

When we are honestly using our gift, though, steeped in the process of truly Being, then we are beautiful to the planet. If we can achieve this as a species, harmony ensues. Alas, a boy can again dream.

If it isn't obvious yet what the role of the holistic athlete is, and how each of our individual bodies connects some important dots in all this, then there's your meditation to keep reading. It's the purpose of this book. In the meantime, be you. It's what you should be best at.

3. Purpose

I'm about to commit what William K. Wimsatt and Monroe C. Beardsley call the Intentional Fallacy, where the author creates his own press release within the book itself by discussing the fervent (and they would argue superfluous) purpose for the creation of said book. Compared to, say, Milton, who wrote that he was "justifying the ways of god to man," my little bit of personal insight here isn't quite as grand, although, at least for myself, it is just as important.

My first book began as a nugget of an idea about 15 years ago, then popped out of my computer as a done deal about 5 years later. As time is notorious for doing, things have changed. With that change comes, well, change. Guess what's amazing about self-publishing a book? You're bamboozled into believing you have complete control over it. You believe that, unlike the tactile arts that exist in permanent display once an artist designates them as finished, this malleable, printable format can be added to or subtracted from at your whim. You own it. You still have the original. You can make a new PDF and send it to the printer whenever you feel the original ideas need tweaking.

What a bunch of crap. The only one owned is the writer. The book, this collection of ideas and dreams, and the transfer of energy from noggin to papyrus, is entirely in control, the writer being forever the minion of the book's whim. I want to change it? No, it's the book that demands it.

The words rule, not who created them.

Some of those words didn't want to be there anymore, others wanted to join the party. An entirely new writing had to rise from the ashes of the old, and here we are.

One word in particular demands better representation. It appears quite a few times in this book, and yet, since my original book launched free thought into the world of movement and strength about a decade ago, this particular word has some folks upset and others laughing, and a few just going 'ewwww.'

This word is to some an uncontrolled industry that is the hyped-up evolution of the traveling medicine shows. This word is late night infomercials, 'celebrity trainers,' and money-sucking useless gadgets. This word means some bad things to really good people, but it wasn't always that way. This word has truer meaning. This word needs to make a comeback.

This word, groggy from mistreatment, mishandling, misrepresentation, misplacement, and misbehaving, is Fitness.

To define where we're going, we'd better define fitness. While we're at it, the word Strength better get some contemplative time in our head space as well. At BodyTribe, and in our workshops and clinics across the country, my clients and students are instructed to define these words. We can't teach, learn, or achieve what isn't defined, but you and I have complete freedom to create the definition.

Let's take it back. Let's make the word Fitness relevant again, no longer the butt of a joke or something to dread (or just boring copy on someone's website). We might have to ignore what gets done in its name, what nonsense happens under its exploited banner. The Fitness Industrial Complex is a bit of a sham, to be sure. But we're not dealing with an industry. We're dealing with you. What does fitness mean to you, and therefore, why is it important?

And, of course, what does Strength mean? Don't worry, we've got some ideas on this one to get you thinking.

The 4 Aspects of Training

No matter how immersed you are in this world of training, whether teacher or student, trainer or client, byproduct of years of propaganda or a veteran only to free thought and exploration, the dubious job of changing any life through movement could be quartered into sections of equal importance:

> Technique
> Program Design
> Personality
> Purpose.

If you recognize this list as the Who, What, How and Why of training, you're perceptive, as I knew you would be. Here's a minor run down of each category...

Personality: The Who. Motivation, support, leadership. The personality might show itself in the vibrancy and enthusiasm of an entire community, yelling about the beauty in their particular brand of pain, or it might be the volume of a single person, so loud that it strips you of any need to think for yourself.

Technique: The How. Short term considerations: the safest, most effective goal oriented movement. Not always "efficient." Long term thoughts: longevity of body. In other words... do it right or suffer the consequences. Maybe not today, but give it time, my friend... give it time.

Program Design: The What. Goal oriented movement selection and execution. What path is going to provide to best outcome?

Purpose: The WHY! The big missing component in a great deal of modern training, and (here's hoping) the most important take-away from this book.

The tenacity of the Fitness Industrial Complex can overwhelm even the brightest of brains, blurring the one aspect of that list that holds all the others accountable. See, without Purpose, the rest simply don't matter. Oh, but therein lies a problem...

Unless we can make the conscious decision to ignore the great juggernaut of the fitness industry, no matter how deep we are in this movement and strength world, we'll have no idea how to formulate the Why. In other words, most folks are lost when setting actual fitness goals.

Hey, it's not that folks are stupid or lacking goal setting skills (at least not you, gentle reader). No, instead our blurry mission is due to being hamstrung in spirit, being thwarted in mission, by a culture of anti-movement, and the profiting thereof. We can only create goals based on experience; therefore, while coming out of the gates towards a fitness goal, the general population is caught in a net of fitness marketing. The Fitness Industrial Complex is founded on this mission statement:

You are ugly. We can help.

As perpetual propaganda, how is someone on this journey, whether new to it or not, going to have any experience in true fitness goal setting? To be blunt, the majority of people stepping into a gym will have one big, fat, wallet-emptying goal:

Please make me more fuckable.

There is nothing wrong with that. Who doesn't want to be desirable? What, though, might humans desire in each other more than body parts and what the eye can take in (or nose, mouth... you get the idea)? Strength. Don't shake your head at me, child, the epitome of attractiveness is strength... at least to anyone who matters. Hold on... hold on! What the heck is

Strength?

I'll explain the process of defining it in a bit. Now here's a story of what might happen when you do:

Not too long ago I was spending time with some friends at Agoge Fitness in lovely Birmingham, Alabama. After a weekend of intensity, movement, and other general physical subculture mayhem, I posed that question to them: what is strength? Eventually we filled up a dry erase board with a collection of answers that had little to do with picking up something heavy, although overcoming obstacles seemed to be a major theme. Words like integrity, perseverance, respect, and understanding filled this board as representations or displays of strength... what it means to be strong. Love topped the list, as it should.

Therefore, if those are the definitions of Strength, then what is strength TRAINING? I'm guessing you don't need it spelled out for you. Be strong, my friends! Somebody who embraces strength, true strength as defined by my kin in Alabama and at most of the workshops I've had the honor of teaching, is far, FAR more... how shall we say it? Fuckable.

Is there anything truly more attractive than simply being an amazing human being, capable of strength in its many forms? Be an important and integral part of your Tribe. Set your goals accordingly. If your trainer/gym/workout partner isn't helping you with this... find one who will. As a trainer, if you're not helping your clients with this... better figure out how. That is step one of our Purpose... and nothing else matters until this is achieved.

We'll chat about some quick tips for defining your journey (goal setting). It is a simple, but demanding process.

First, as promised, define the words Strength and Fitness. These are the two real goals of movement practice (weight loss and aesthetic changes are a byproduct and will go on a separate list of goals).

This rant begs the question of where the heck am I

going?

Let's accept that to fully begin our own personal philosophies, we must embrace a metaphysical component to our training. Of course a huge part of this book is the reiteration of this idea of embodiment, so worry not... you'll be reminded constantly. In fact, if you're expecting an actual physical program offered anywhere in this book, you'll have better chance with any other of the 1500 books about training that have come out this year. The What and How are ubiquitous. Every article, video, book and podcast are replete with what to do and how to do it.

But, as mentioned earlier, the What and How are empty sans the Why. That's the real work. The painful work, way more than the toil the iron demands from us. Our souls are requesting something more.

We have a simple trick to defining these words, Strength and Fitness, although 'simple' is not synonymous with 'easy.' Ask yourself why they're important. Boom... you have your definition. Oh, and you may discover that Strength and Fitness share underlying principles in your metaphysical pursuit, practically being synonymous. Of course they would.

4. The Relationship

As development, health, and longevity are the rewards of obeying the laws of man's mechanism, so degeneracy, disease, and premature death are no less the legitimate punishment of their violation.

Whatever will secure the greatest degree of strength, vigor, health, and perfection of the physical organization, should be adopted and applied by all, as the first and most important duty of life.
- David P. Butler, <u>The Lifting Cure</u>, 1868

Training is not servitude. Others do not impose training on us. Training is a direct vehicle of our practice of mindfulness. Our training is for those who embrace a journey of true empowerment, both for themselves and their tribe.

Life is suffering. Overcoming is living. Finding it fun is truly being alive!

To paraphrase Thich Nhat Hanh, we can learn how to go home to our bodies. Through mindfulness in our movements and intensity, a dialog presents itself between us and our bodies. Can we listen to and understand the language of our body? The dialog often isn't what the mind is telling us.

Is it really a surprise that the relationships with our bodies aren't... well... good? Heck, in many cases they're not there at all beyond our tenuous idea of the body being submissive to our whims. "Body, get me to the fridge!" What we're witnessing in the proliferation of diseases and the damage of our personal ecosystems is simple mutiny.

With a smidgen of awareness, and a scoop of mindfulness, it will dawn on us how little we listen.

We command.
We demand.
We expect.
We damage.
We decorate.
We subvert.
We ignore.

We don't listen. We also slather the feedback with a heap of cognitive dissonance. The results, therefore, are blamed on everything but our own choices.

Bummer, since we have a best friend and lifelong companion with us at all times. Our little flesh packets aren't just our vessels, but living, feeling, talking machines that, although I'm currently addressing them as separate units, are actually very much US!

I posit a bold premise. Our relationships with our bodies, ourselves, will be the precedent for all of our relationships. Suddenly the cliché of having to love yourself before you can love others has a potent ring to it, doesn't it?

THAT'S what authentic training is - fully grokking your relationship with your body. The fitness industry is failing in not recognising this. It has actually done a swell job of creating an even greater rift between us and our bodies, giving us false ideas of harmony and balance. The industry has convinced us that our brains know our bodies better than our bodies do. That's a dangerous understanding and has a huge effect on our tribes.

Not far from me lives a growing thinking being, too young to be legend, too unfamiliar to be iconic, who roams the nearby wilderness, both industrial and natural, with a fluidity in skill and the whisper of true stealth, complete with the child's grasp of curiosity and wonder. He dreams big, holding himself to a high standard while hoping the rest of us might join him. His relationship with his body is profound and tribal, and always growing. In his own words, he speaks of how we are what we do, and we can only do as much as we are. Meet Victor, and until he writes his own book, I'll quote him liberally.

We are vascular, veins everywhere. Scars from epic adventures, challenges, and training. Eyes that spot wild edibles, poisonous plants, animals, weather patterns, hidden routes, interactions, habits, emotion, truth, river currents, materials for tools, shelters, weak points in a place's defense, and so much more. Ears that hear secrets of the earth. A nose that smells more and processes more information than most people do in their entire essence. Legs that can run very fast and very far; that can leap and kick and lift and squeeze and balance with perfection; that are built, maintained, and fed distance, speed, steep ascents, and opponents on a regular basis. Dependable, reliable. Lungs that allow you to haul ass for long periods of time; lungs that hold tons of air as you dive deeper and deeper. Callused and thick-skinned hands with the grip of a pitbull's bite; dense knuckles; hands that can wield a blade with skill; hands that can handle hot objects and thorns without getting injured. Bones like spring steel; dense, strong, flexible, dangerous. Feet that sneak with no sound, that can carry you miles unshod, spring you along with power for endless mileage.

A body familiar with distance, harsh winds, cold rains, storms, steep rock, sharp thorns, high walls, big drops, large gaps, burning roads and rooftops, strong opponents, high pressure depths, high altitudes and thin air, roasting sun, freezing river and lake depths, slippery mud, long rope, rough cable, swaying heights, the steepness of mountains, the

darkness of subterranean chambers and moonless nights, the
grueling weight of another person/ruck, the stress of necessity
during emergency, and the roughness of combat.
We are rugged from use. We do not seek a stage. We do not
seek acceptance. We do not seek fame. We seek strength. We
seek awareness. Freedom. We might not dance or trick all that
well, but we can kick ass and get places most people can't. We
are the true ninjas, the ones who know the trails, at night,
underwater, cold or hot, underground, high above, unseen...
Our tools are obtained and maintained for use, not display.
This is the way of the scout.

Look at a mountain or explore it? Look at a river or
swim it? Settle down or go exploring? Hide from and complain
about the elements or thrive in them? Fill your lives with
excuses against or fill your lives with reasons for? Don't have
time or don't make time?

Slum Lords, Slave Drivers and Slow Poisoners.

The not so divine comedy these days is how, with our
vast intellects, we choose ignorance. Imagine the consequences
if we couldn't quite get away with that choice as easily. What if
we were more transparent? Literally. What if we were see-
through? If our innards were as visible as our outer flesh
packet, only hidden by clothing, what would the result be? Not
unlike the several body-on-display shows that have been
touring the country for a while, what if our living internal
machines were transparent and always visible, providing an
open book of consequences of our choices for anyone to see?
What would the social awareness of this blatant feedback
aesthetic be? Are we a little less likely to abuse our systems to
our current extent if our insides spoke simply by being visible?
Would we be so quick to light up if our blackened lungs stared
out at the world daily? Perhaps we'd be slower on the prefab
cardboard foods if our transparency revealed the state of our

arteries. I'm guessing visible large proportions of visceral adipose tissue would be considered less than sexy.

A quick trip to Doctor Snipsnip and a big bowl of cognitive dissonance are our current quick fixes for what ails our self esteems, so if veiling our poor choices were more of a challenge, would the 'medical' field simply be an anatomy factory, cranking out new innards for anyone with the ducats to swap old for new?

Or would we start to give a darn about ourselves, if at least to avoid public ridicule?

"Check out the nice open coronary arteries on her," comments the construction worker between catcalls. "I'd like to feel the contractile impulse of THAT sinoatrial node!"

Wanna know what the heart or lungs or spleen do? Sure you do. A pox on the brittle-minded college student who wandered into the Bodies Revealed show scowling "ewww, this is gross." Sorry, child, but that's YOU, or at least a chemically preserved dead representation of you.

Who's to Blame?

Modifying beliefs to be in line with one's actions sure seems easier than the inverse. The shining examples of this may be in ill treatment towards others. "To treat badly another person whom we consider a reasonable human being," writes James Loewen, in Lies My Teacher Told Me, "creates a tension between act and attitude that demands resolution. We cannot erase what we have done and to alter our future behavior may not be in our interest. To change our attitude is easier. Suddenly our behavior is justified toward that person, who may be a loved one, friend or simply just a decent human being, because we can change our attitude about them quicker and easier then we can change ourselves."

Loewen considers this an example of cognitive dissonance, which is often defined as a psychological phenomenon which refers to the discomfort felt as a discrepancy between what you already know or believe, and new information or interpretation. Consider how often, on small scales (the original concept was applied to cults and deep, massive brainwashing), we are capable of this daily.

Is it far fetched, then, to accept that we often apply this concept internally, not just changing our beliefs to meet our actions towards others, instead changing our beliefs to match how we treat ourselves? If the good person we are mistreating happens to be our self, then what do we have to believe about ourselves to justify this behavior? A popular behavior is to glorify the mistreatment, and this misplaced value comes in two common flavors I. The first I refer to as the Bukowski Syndrome, thinking that our self-destructive behaviors are the romantic means to artistic ends; our suffering then becomes beautiful martyrdom for art's sake. A dangerous chunk of my creative peer group suffers from this. C'mon, even Bukowski quit drinking at some point. A mantra to my groovy artist friends: If Tom Waits can give up smoking, so can you.

The second version is that we simply start to believe we deserve our self-abuse; that we are, indeed, crap and therefore no amount of crap we ingest or partake in is too bad for us. A less severe version of this self-denial is simply believing a weakness about ourselves that we haven't the strength to overcome. The phrase "I can't help it" might start as a cute justification early on, but if the behavior continues, it becomes a destructive mantra.

What might start as a glorification, where vice becomes a reward ('I deserve this because I'm good') will eventually change to abuse if the behavior and its consequences continues ('I deserve this because I'm bad'). This type of cognitive dissonance is, of course, found in degrees, a complete spectrum from small binges to big addictions, slight eating and diet changes to full blown eating disorders. In fact, even something with good intentions like a 'diet' could be illogical in the face of truth. Well-honed, time-honored marketing techniques can sure shake our reasoning skills.

Cognitive dissonance also says that the more struggle or sacrifice made in coming to a belief, the stronger that belief will be and the less likely one is to concede to being wrong, even in the face of blatant evidence to the contrary (read: truth). This justification is why the current anti-science of the modern fitness industry continues to perpetuate so many myths. The woman who spends 90 minutes on the stair climber every day for years will have a much harder time stepping off, even if positive change hasn't occurred to her body for months. The bodybuilder who spends hours training his biceps will justify his quest for vanity by somehow convincing himself that, since weight training is healthy, those hours spent striving for massive beefcake status are somehow good for him.

Thanks to layers to cognitive dissonance that some meathead like myself won't even begin to pontificate on, we reach no simple answers or antidotes. Perhaps we can each take a look at what type of potentially (or blatantly) destructive behavior we may heap upon ourselves, or others, and ask if such behavior really fits into what we believe at our core. We need to question ourselves on occasion. It's okay; we're not 'wrong,' but we're not above self-evaluation either. See what you come up with.

With this strong campaign for disconnection from our bodies always looming, what can we do? First, identify the culprit. Most of us will fall into at least one of these three categories.

The Slave Driver: We'll discuss this in more depth further on, but this category involves the brain as the control center, believing it knows best. Duped through external or internal sources, the brain believes that punishment of the body, in our context through the guise of fitness, is a satisfying bondage. Pain and suffering, masquerading as training, are the foundations of the Slave Driver's personal relationship between brain and body.

The Slow Poisoner: We all eat wrong. Vegan? Wrong. Paleo? Wrong. Blood, bone and bile diet? Wrong, wrong, wrong. It will only take you 30 seconds on the internet to learn that. It's no wonder we throw our hands up and say 'to hell with it... hand me the uber-spicy deep fried corn mush product that turns our hands and face into a color that can only be described as Oompa-Loompa orange.

When an argument can be made for or against any way of eating, and with Amazon telling me there are 224,479 diet books available (really), is it surprising more of us aren't cannibals, so confused from the overload of information that we just decided to eat our own kind? Far be it for this book to tread on already well-worn territory. Suffice to say, we're a nation of slow poisoners.

Midtown Sacramento is blessed with a few weekly farmer's markets, plus the Natural Foods Co-op, which we'll use as one end of the spectrum of grocery choices. Then, within short driving distance, we have 6 large chain grocery stores. Moving down the spectrum we have over two dozen corner marts, drug stores, and gas station mini-marts. With some quick math in my head, of the available food stuffs to purchase in my neighborhood that aren't restaurants, that's probably about 80-90% packaged, processed, pre-fab junk.

In our westernized land of easily accessible packaged poison, the challenge of having a decent relationship with how we fuel our bodies will be a constant struggle. Just remember a motto we'll repeat throughout this book:

You matter. Treat yourself accordingly.

The Slum Lord: Your body is barely a consideration. It gets less attention than your car, which you won't even lift a finger for until something on the dashboard flashes red or it simply stops running. For whatever reason, this relationship between mind and body disappeared years ago. Maybe, just maybe, you'll pay attention when the tenants start bitching enough or the foundation cracks... but probably not.

These relationship archetypes thrive in a culture of personal relationship dysfunction. I'm hoping we can be ambassadors for some change, because the fitness industrial complex is not offering the help it claims to, sometimes feeding the dysfunctions more than fixing them.

5. The 85%.
Or How the Industry Is
Failing As and What
We Can Do About It.

I'm calling out the Fitness Industrial Complex, and I'm saying it is failing. Not in profit making, but in everything else.

One big reason: its recruiting program stinks.

My buddy Dave Hall will drop this bomb on us: only about 15% of our culture is participating in movement and fitness. Kevin Geary says only about 1% succeed at making it a lifetime of good choices. Although that second number seems hard to prove, it still behooves us to ask what the heck is going on here.

I admit to once having a bias in believing that everyone had access to proper movement education. My travels and wanderings, which find me teaching (and learning!) all over this country, have made blatant a strong, and contrary, truth. With just a quick glance, it is easy to see how the fitness industrial complex is actually failing in its recruitment program, if there could be a case that such a program exists. All I needed for proof of this failure was to spend time with my family.

My brilliant, wonderful kin are part of the 85%, therefore the usual online offerings of, oh, just about any website or video channel (including my own) isn't going to do much to help them begin their journey. The fitness industry as a whole has no proper welcome wagon, instead believing that shiny new toys or flashy programs are the answer to recruiting the non-movers. Nope. Not quite.

This insight isn't news. History has shown us that once a social movement becomes an industry, its tenets become products, and that rarely turns out well. So how does the Fitness Industrial Complex actually disconnect us from our bodies? Glad you asked.

First, we screw things up by thinking that movement and exercise are synonymous. Exercise is simply movement as a task towards a reward. Therein lies the problem. Our society thrives on being as busy as possible, which is not synonymous with productive, but sure looks the part. We sink a lot of faith into the concept of sacrifice. Life becomes a simple, yet busy, system of sacrifice and reward, and we become convinced that movement should be no different. Hence we believe that the rewards from movement must only come through struggle and suffering, just like everything else. Fun just isn't part of the equation.

We believe that the greater the suffering, the greater the reward. No wonder, as a culture, we abhor exercise.

Yup, the fitness industry is actually pretty poor at teaching movement. It's too quick to promote exercise!

We really do need to trash this entire industry and start over. Let this be a call out to trainers and coaches, and perhaps anyone buying into the current system: please stop feeding the machine, that broken process of just teaching exercise. Find the joy in movement, maybe on your own, or by being a guide through someone's discovery of their own potential.

Here is a fresh idea: What if we actually taught and promoted the ability to listen to the body?

The first big step in any relationship is the ability to listen. Then the dialog begins by replacing judgment with compassion, maybe even with an understanding that would empower the 15% as well as the 85%. Those of us who have bought into the fitness scene are quite tempted to call non-movers lazy or scared. How about another theory?

Bodies understand movement better than brains. Brains, though, are what created the fitness industry. Brains believe what the industry has taught them movement is supposed to look like (and how much it should cost). If bodies thought for themselves, so to speak, how do you think they'd perceive what we call 'fitness?' Under the assumption that your body would even want to go to a gym, what would that gym look like? The shiny spectacle of the common chain gyms would have NO appeal to your body. Cardio theaters and color-coded 'strength' equipment are brain candy, but bodies would reject them. Even dingy warehouses with nothing but some bars, bumpers, and a pull-up station would seem sort of dull. Maybe anything under a roof would seem antithetical to the body's mission of movement and exploration.

Our bodies want what we used to call recess. Intensity in fun, challenging forms, and the brain and body have differing opinions of what this looks like. So my theory is that at least some of the 85% might simply be hearing the muffled cries of their bodies screaming at the fitness industry: "What the hell is that crap? That's not what I want!" Don't write them off as lazy... maybe just perceptive, but lacking real resources.

In my videos and workshops, I ramble on about the child's mind, this archetypal consciousness where movement is understood, if not completely consciously, to be integral to all processes of the self. Therefore approaching movement as a perpetual student creates greater potential for growth. The child-like approach to movement is curious, creative, explorational, and judgment-free. Although the fitness industry does a fine job of treating us like children, nothing about the industry's presentation actually appeals to the child-like approach our bodies desire.

Our adult brains buy into a culture that tries to squelch play somewhere around high school, turning movement into a series of categories, formulas and routines geared towards a superficial product. Maybe some of that 85% are still tuned into their child-like selves and can simply sense that this isn't what the body actually needs.

Yes, laziness does exist. Just not physically. Laziness is a brain game; another version of the disconnect from the body. Many friends of mine claim they suffer from laziness. They're a peer group of artists, parents, writers, professors, musicians... quite productive in many aspects of their lives. They're not lazy. They're scared. They suffer a disconnect from their bodies and have yet to be shown the value of movement, or a venue or outlet for which their body finds it appealing to begin the journey.

This disconnection is a bummer. Because all of their current productivity will cease as soon as their bodies give out. Their tribes – families, peers groups, jobs, communities – will lose an important member. The body doesn't want this. It isn't lazy. Possibly poorly fueled and tired, but not without the essential desire to participate in life.

There is a deep psychology in movement, or lack thereof, which brings us to a huge point...

Our culture has a fear of movement. The fitness industry does more to perpetuate that fear that aleve it. Prescribed exercise is now about avoiding movement rather than enjoying it.

The industry is nothing but brains selling to other brains, not bodies being heard. Movement is being sold as categories, sections, and trends. From 'cardio' to mobility, Zumba to CrossFit, movement has been turned into pieces, parts, and genres. The caveat is that body doesn't think that way. Although some structure helps us reach goals, dogma can get in the way. Chosen places, correct times, and approved movements are doing more to turn movement into a stressFUL experience, the exact opposite of what movement is supposed to do. Disconnecting us from our bodies. Antithetical to a true relationship we all need.

Some of that might be the built-in politics of an industry.

First, if we have an industry, we have leaders. Leaders have followers. None of this will truly breed a fun-filled stomping ground for the body. My Facetube feed is filled with industry posts geared towards trainers about being an 'industry leader.' Here's the problem...

A tribe can usually only handle a few leaders, but can have many, many teachers. A leader has followers. A teacher has students. How many followers can become leaders? Very few. How many students can become teachers? All of them.

The 15% better get off our self-centered asses and recognize our potential teacher status. Since every true teacher is perpetually a student, we've got to shoulder that empowering responsibility as well. Are you game?

A mountainous chunk of the info bouncing around right now – the youface videos, the articles on superbadass.org and bloodWOD.gov - is the 15% talking to each other. Heck, it might be happening right here, right now. And that's groovy, since our tribe needs to share, educate, and support each other (The three needs of a tribe: communication, equality, and sustainability. More on that later).

Industry media tip: the phenomenon of saturating social media with our workouts, silly people tricks, and feats of superhuman strength sure isn't attracting that 85%. Trainers trying to impress other trainers might be more turn-off than seduction.

Any campaign that is currently in place to entice the non-moving population is more flawed than the North Carolina legislature's idea of "tolerance."

If you happen to be a trainer, then you also need to be a mentor for goal setting. Not our goals, theirs. Our job is to show them what is possible. We're allowed to jump and play and laugh and love and dance and sing and rage and climb and fall and swoon and crave and fly. Allowed? We're supposed to. It is what the body is made for. Consider not denying it.

One of the biggest lessons? Better choices now for more choices later... because the inverse is also true.

I wanna tell everyone they're beautiful and strong, and I want to start with you. Plans and programs and charts and levels and structure might be clinically proven but what about a simple hello and an open door policy to shine? That might be what the 85% need to get their party started.

6. Protect, Provide, Play

How did you answer the earlier question of why this stuff is important? Maybe it becomes more obvious, as we get deeper into this book, that training can (heck, *should*) mean a bit more than a physical practice -that the ripples of our strength can spread wide through our humanness. This observation should have become a bit blatant when you decided to ask 'why is this stuff important?' Your purpose, if I were to garner a guess, began to emerge.

In fact, I'm betting that your Purpose extends significantly beyond you. It quite possibly includes your relationship with your tribes, and how you can be a more integral part of them. This becomes a two-part lesson.

First, you now have a true, profound journey ahead of you. Second, your discerning eyes may notice that big chunks of your current program actually don't really support your purpose. For instance, my purpose has three major components, Protect, Provide and Play. If my training isn't supporting this purpose trilogy, then I have to ask myself some questions about why I'm doing what I'm doing.

Protect

What is the role of peace? Not an easy question to answer, since the ideal and the reality suffer some discrepancies between them. For instance, it takes a pretty drastic lifestyle change to 'rest in peace.' The annals of history seem to support this turn of phrase, as in the only way we, as a species, will ever truly be at peace is when we're all gone. Globally, peace seems to simply mark the small gaps of time between conflicts, meaning it is fleeting, if it exists at all. Recent human history doesn't offer a single time when we were ever, as a planet, at peace, so maybe peaceful resting will only arrive, as I hinted in an earlier chapter (and like the idiom suggests), when we're all dead.

As compassionate beings we can adopt a pacifist[1] ideology in our hearts and spirits, since it's a swell idea to at least want an end to global conflict. But there are good reasons to cultivate the body of a warrior, and the role of protector.

Our industrial complex society sets up our community, economy, and political machine for constantly preparing for war. Violent conflict seems the inevitable conclusion of our very structure. It can seem as if nothing in our politics seems in place for preparing us for peace, since it is completely understood that peace for our culture is a short term, passing fad, simply the time between battles.

> *"...perhaps the most extraordinary result of nuclear technology is that it has brought the human race as a whole to the point at which physical and spiritual salvation are no longer separable. It is no longer possible to save our skin while remaining ignorant of our own motives and unconscious of our own cultures."*

> - M. Scott Peck, M.D., The Different Drum

Is our way, our 'human nature,' that of conflict? Well, of course, and we'll chat about this more in a bit. Suffering seems to be a key ingredient in every philosophical or theological stew. Overcoming obstacles is hardwired in our software to achieve humanness.

---

[1] Despite the word having a bit of a homophonic relationship with the word 'passive,' pacifism can be a powerful, active, and potent form of human rights advocacy. Hating war isn't synonymous with fearing battle.

Conflict through domination, i.e. war, seems to arise, like Emerson's quote about industry, from a lengthened shadow of one person. There always seems to be one (or a small handful) leading many towards this domination quest. War, despite whatever government creates it, is rarely democratic.

The role of Protector, though, extends beyond the cliché of Steven Seagal movies. Bullies manifest beyond human greed, even beyond physical, even tactile form. From elements to emotions, from the destructive force of a tornado to the devastation of clinical loneliness, the foes of our tribes might not always be in the form of martial combat. My training needs direct application to being a dependable protector. How about yours?

In a healthy tribe, attention is divided equally, making wealth less important and domination a low priority. Culturally, we've never experienced a scenario where security is guaranteed and attention is blanketed amongst all, so we don't know if someone would still have the need to try to dominate a culture even in an ideally healthy scenario.

The question therefore exists: are we, by nature, 'good,' or simply 'polite' due to possible consequences? Heck, maybe we all have true potential for the vilest of power conflicts and evil deeds, but it takes so much damn work and we're simply too damn lazy.

Pax Exerceo

Exerceo: to train, cultivate, keep at work, exercise, practice.

Pax Exerceo. Peace through training. This concept is my daydream, which acknowledges that peace is not a total lack of conflicts. Instead peace becomes the GOAL of the conflicts; accepting smaller conflicts as lessons in communication or tribal empowerment so the major conflicts become unnecessary. Can a quest for strength and ability play a role in this admitted unreal fantasy?

How can it not?

Kant mentioned that our belief in God was moot, since it would behoove us to behave as if there was one regardless. In other words, let's be nice to each other, without having to base it on a concept of rewards and punishments. Then why? As Perry Farrell[2] wrote, just because. That's how I'd like to approach peace. I'd like to attempt it, whether it is realistic or not, just because.

During a recent training session, I caught myself in deep rumination during a pre-squat ritual. I was almost obscenely caressing a barbell before putting it on my back. I twisted it, tugged at it, and gripped the piss out of it, all the while knowing I was going to lift it. During my pre-squat dance, I noticed that I had help. Often I lift alone during the fairly quiet time at BodyTribe, early in the afternoon when people who actually do important things are at work. This day was different, finding the battle between gravity and me in a much more public scenario, later in the afternoon surrounded by multiple wars/parties going on around me. I was slow to understand the process, but by my last set, some magic began sinking in, and the barbell and I connected, no longer a battle but a celebration. My tribe was there to help.

I'm obtuse, but not totally oblivious. Around my squat cage bubble was hard work. Demons being slayed, angels being embraced, hateful regimes being toppled, and bridges of opportunity being built, all within the other cages and platforms and mats around me. The Tribe was alive with strength, and before I knew it, I was inspired. My bar knew it, my legs knew it, and eventually my consciousness caught up.

---

[2] The man who, among other notable things, brought the word Lollapalooza into our modern lexicon. Quick, off-topic trivia: 1) The word came from a Three Stooges movie. 2) Did you remember that Siouxie and the Banshees were part of the original tour lineup? Love them.

Webster has this to say about the word "athlete:" Anyone trained to contend in exercises requiring great physical agility and strength; one who has great activity and strength; a champion. Our little power dojo was spilling over with athletes. I saw a room of champions, even if most of them haven't competed on any public stage. No quest for celebrity status, and no worship of corporate logo sponsors going on this night. Instead there was a hive of activity, brutal and playful. This iron war dance wasn't for fame, bragging rights, scholarships or medals. What I witnessed this evening, and experience everyday with my tribe, is the winning of battles against personal foes. Overcoming these obstacles will lock the door against laziness, and if small tribes like ours can do it, maybe the big tribe has a chance. Our heroes are us, learning to protect ourselves from sloth and decline. I train to protect that.

Provide.

I get to assist people in becoming stronger. My role may not be much more than simply pulling up a seat to watch a comedy/drama/thriller/documentary about a growing relationship between someone and their body, but on occasion, when the credits roll, there's BodyTribe listed as, if not the director, then at least the gaffer, or assistant to the grip, proof that we got to somehow be part of the show, the star-studded extravaganza that we'll call You.

I point and grunt something instructive and somehow that eventually translates into a more capable member of the tribe. If only I were that magical... truth is all the work came from you, but us pointers and grunters at BodyTribe are sure glad to be part of your journey.

A premise has grown in my little trainer brain from being in the center of so much purposeful flux, which I mentioned previously. The relationship between a person and their body that we keep yammering about has a direct correlation with that person and their other relationships (interpersonal, spiritual, intellectual, etc.). Oh, I won't wax ridiculous about this now, but the glaring story around these parts is the relationship between folks and our tribe. What good is strength and ability if it doesn't mean the strength and ability of the tribe?

The strange coincidence of the week, which I'll expose in a moment, needs prefacing. My writing style, as obviously brilliant, enlightening, and humble as it is, doesn't flow out of me like a stream of genius. In fact, I have to reach into my bag of tricks in phases, with a lot of painful pauses during the writing process. These time gaps are filled with food preparation, making baby talk to the closest animal, pacing around pretending I'm not watching last night's Daily Show episode on the internet, or reading what other people write, all to make it seem like these breaks are intentional, when in reality, my said bag of tricks is simply empty.

Today, in between one of the above paragraphs, I decided to reread one of Dave Draper's old newsletters. Take a look:

> The obvious truth is you and I take care of ourselves so we are more able to take care of those around us. We are extraordinarily generous and considerate people, like a breed of our own. We lift weights that we may lighten the load for our neighbors. We eat healthy foods that we may care for the ill when they grow faint. We seek longevity because someone must attend the aging and failing in their time of need. We sleep, rest and relax with peace-loving diligence that we may serve others tirelessly. We, through our consistent exercise, develop discipline, patience and compassion, needed character qualities when called upon by God and man to mitigate strife and negotiate peace.

See? I can't even paraphrase that and call it my own, like I usually do.

Our relationship with our health and the ability of our bodies translates to the relationship we have with other aspects of our lives. The one artistic license I might call Dave on is that he stated it was obvious. He's an optimist. I see it as something that COULD happen, but there is no guarantee. Keep an eye open for it. Having a defined purpose helps.

7. USEFUL

If all human lives depended upon their usefulness - as might be judged by certain standards - there would be a sudden and terrific mortality in the world.
- Gene Tunney

Useful. Valuable. Boring sounding, yet we sure give it a lot of energy, at least as a culture, but we fake it as individuals. We're busy *looking* busy, but busy doesn't mean useful.

Am I useful?

We're so busy appearing busy that we don't actually get much done. As a nation we LOVE being useful. No, wait... we love *appearing* useful. We'll throw so much money, energy, and hyperbole into a cause or project, but usually a productive outcome is more of a surprise than a planned result.

Did that stink of pessimism? Sorry. There is good work being done, to be sure, but let's face it, we're usually just busy appearing busy.

Did you just say I look a bit taller? It's this extra large soapbox I've just climbed up on. I can see your house from up here. Good time to do burpees... training at high elevations is supposed to do wonders for your superhero powers.

E-Bazon, FaceTube and YouBook are home to thousands of books, videos, and websites willing to offer you the keys to the How and What of fitness and strength. Heck, it's a big part of my bread and butter. I think I even have a Tweety account, or some such thing, and my beautiful (but gassy) dog Scarlet even has her own Instagram account[3] (make me my millions, sweetheart!). As we keep pointing out in this book, a big vacuum exists where the Why should be. A truth no one wants to face: if we confront the why behind our decisions, fitness or otherwise, many of our choices seem... well... sorta dumb. If your keen eye takes a gander through any corporate gym, you'll see what I mean.

Am I useful? Oh, there it is again. It's a funny question, isn't it? Annoying, like a redundant poke from a 6-year old's snot-covered index finger in your rib cage. Ouch. Stop it. Ouch. Enough already!

Perhaps it's annoying because it's THE question. It's a less sugarcoated way of asking if you're a good person, or a just person, or a caring person. That's what being useful is... gettin' shit done to benefit the tribe. But we sorta hide from asking if our actions or lifestyle will prove useful because... well, it's tricky isn't it?

Yes or No, True or False. Yikes... for once you finally want to answer in essay form.

This topic has been sitting in my spiritual in-box for months now, and I haven't posed the question because I'm a bit nervous of my own answer.

Am I useful? If this test question were a bit more multiple choice than True/False, I'd pick the third box:

"Unsure"

Next to it I might scribble "but am working on it."

---

[3] www.instagram.com/scarletonmymind.

8. Play
(or Why Grown Ups are So Flippin' Boring)

According to Daniel Dumbrowski, the ancient Greeks liked play. It was important enough to be foundational in their idealized concepts of all things human. Play to them had three faces, Frolic, Competition, and War, and the second two categories had a far greater purity to them than what we perceive them to mean today.

Competition was play within guidelines and rules, the goal being for all competitors to grow, learn, and increase their awareness and understanding. That resembles our current idea of competition as much as the first Clash of the Titans movie resembled the recent remake. The distorted modern ideal of competition is completely about winning, usually winning at any cost. It's domination of something or someone. For the Greeks, that is an entirely different category: War.

Ever jump in a leaf pile? That's Frolic. It begins when we giggle as babies for no reason other than joy. In fact, to say frolic = joy would not earn anything below an A in the algebra of life.

Stuart Brown, who studies play... he's a play scientist, which might be the coolest job in the world... discusses play, with the emphasis on the quality of frolic, as being essential to our development, but not just as snot-nosed pre-adults. Our relationship with the planet, with each other, and with ourselves, all benefit from the lessons we learn from play. Within nature, play is an altered state, a bit like LSD for the spirit, which allows us to explore what is possible.

Absence of play, according to the experts, makes us crazy. Gonzo. Psycho... no, really. People like Stuart Brown, who take play seriously enough to make some science out of it, have found a gaping void where play should be in the formative years of folks who are less than caring about right versus wrong later in life. You know... sociopaths. Yikes. Um... let's go climb a tree.

If we remember Dumbrowski's telling of the ancient Greek model of the three faces of play, the seemingly purposeless movements and interactions of Frolic, to the rule-based pursuit of empowerment of Competition, to the quest for dominance of War, then it ain't hard to make a correlation to our modern strength training practices. The lack of seriousness in Frolic means that it isn't taken very seriously (an ironic correlation that, as mentioned, can make us bat shit crazy). Ironically we'll shout and slap and grunt ourselves silly during training with huge emphasis on the other two aspects

We'll make a pitch here that Play and Movement are the conjoined twins of our training protocol, and let's remember that both of those have the footnote of "*see also: **Strength**"* in their definitions in the BodyTribe dictionary. Therefore our authentic strength model might tarnish if our training is decidedly heavier with any of these three aspects. A good ol' evenly sliced pie chart might be the graphic representation of what we seek between the three faces of play within our training and within our lives. Let any aspect of play dominate your ritual and it's time you examined how you get along with the rest of the planet. Once again, I bet the direct correlation will be apparent.

Frolic is play *seemingly* without purpose... doing just to do, being just to be, moving just to move. Animals and children seem to grasp this, but adults seem to forget it. In fact, legendary fitness and body expert Bonnie Prudden called our adult process of forgetting how to enjoy this level of play as *adulticide*, because forgetting our child self is killing our adult self.

Maybe there is a purpose. It simply may not jive with our adult brains. Frolic contains a recipe that is so subtle, so unconscious, that we forget how integral it is to completing the potential of our DNA. Spontaneity, creativity, and imagination are the bass, drums, and piano that makes up this particular rhythm section, and without that jazz in your soul, your organic machine may as well be a robot.

We're more verb than noun. Our bodies are in constant flux even when we are still. Our minds are in perpetual creation even when we're not thinking. We, despite our best efforts, are constantly trying to BE, even when we put all our efforts into just existing. Purposeful movement, meaning anything voluntary, offers us a chance to understand our relationship with, oh, all sorts of stuff. Ourselves, first and foremost, and, not surprisingly, that usually correlates to your other relationships. Movement and strength are simply indicators of our relationship with our bodies, and our relationship with our bodies is an indicator of our relationship to everything else on the planet. If that relationship isn't playful, what is it? And why? And what does that say about our other relationships?

Therefore frolic has a great deal of purpose. It just doesn't feel like it does. Play increases problem solving. Play is born from curiosity and exploration. Emotional, cognitive, and social behaviors are byproducts of the chaos of frolic, the organization of competition, and the focus of battle. So is, importantly, imagination!

Once again...

You matter. Treat yourself accordingly.

The modern Fitness Industrial Complex is designed for you to be led, for you to obey. Granted, in entertaining ways, like an aggressive stationary cycle class, or sometimes into battle, like a major conflict with a potent minion of gravity, say, a heavily loaded barbell. Unfortunately, we're often having our hand held by some sort of expert, someone who has done the thinking and experiencing for us and can direct us down a path they've already mapped out over geography they have thoroughly charted. You are no longer an explorer, no longer a curious spirit discovering personal limits as much as patron on an amusement ride, following tracks already laid out for you.

Prefab programs lack personal growth. Unless our play-o-meter allows us to let our inner 8-year old see the information as simply Play-doh that we can twist and mash and create something of our own with, we'll end up losing the ultimate lesson. We know nothing until we make it our own.

The trainer/client or teacher/student scenario has the most impact if both parties can understand it more as a master/apprentice scenario, letting a journey unfold that will ultimately turn the person on the receiving end of the info into their own artist, their own master.

Otherwise the lessons are moot.

Play is the discovery of personal limits. As children this is done without awareness or judgment, which on one hand is a freedom, and on the other... well...possible danger. If that isn't a germ for possibility, what is? We can create and expand our brains, muscles, and spirits with only the seed of information, the initial cell of an idea or concept or tool. It is through play that we understand our freedom to make our own journeys with that seed, mold our own empires of fire with just a spark. We need to embrace that freedom as adults, when we're in the position to embrace sagacity as a guide to our search. Instead we often set the limits before we even begin the journey, usually by hiding from free thought, dodging discernment, curiosity, and purity of enthrallment through creation. Adults judge movement. Children do not.

Documenting Play: Oxymoron?

Embodiment disappears when we obsess with external measuring sticks. Heart rate, sets and reps, times intervals... all have a place, but as pieces, not law. Our most life-giving properties, our super software that let's us earn a place on this green globe's scheme, is immeasurable. Spontaneity, creativity... is there a love clock I don't know about? Can you chart my passion on your Droid? Frank Forencich, the Exuberant Animal guru, jokes about giving into the modern trends of documentation and measurement by creating APE (Ancestral Physical Education) units. *"An APE unit is simply a full day of sustained, outdoor locomotion, physicality and exploration: a sunup to sundown effort of moving your body in the natural world."*

Combine your APE units with his Combined Physicality Rating (that's right... CPR), and, he quips...

> *"...We find an ideal solution that should keep everyone happy. By working together, we can create a composite metric that we can log into a spreadsheet and upload into a data base and then get down to some serious, laborious number-crunching. We can work some formulas and write an iPhone app that will help us keep the whole thing on tap for instant reference and comparisons.*
>
> *"Or, we could just go outside and move our bodies. It worked before and it can work again."*

Hey, don't count me out of the counting and tallying clan. Everything we do can have indicative properties. Say what you like about our supposed primitive DNA... we dig comparing stats, often against each other, but most importantly, against ourselves. We thrive on benchmarks. A little hard and fast data at our fingertips can give us linear proof of our previous boundaries crumbling through our efforts. Representing those efforts through some good solid characters and numbers, graphs and charts, can tickle a logical embodiment in us, if understood for what it is... the mapping of the physical process. If we dwell completely in the metaphysical, the touchy-feely quest for movement Nirvana, sans our very human ability to keep track of a few things, then we're actually missing a key ingredient to the Embodiment special sauce.

Therein lies the potential danger of the 'nothing but primal' movement. We're not primal. We're here and now. We need to understand our current relationships. A little tracking and some occasional math is a lubricant to understanding, not an obstacle to it.

The problem is the fitness-world's obsession of finding pure truth in those numbers. They tell us as much about our connection with ourselves as a diagnostic test tells you about the driving experience of your car. Whether the number comes from a scale, the weight on the bar, or the time on a clock, it is not a complete representation of what you can do, of who you are as a moving creature. Heck, in the case of the scale, it tells you diddly squat about your abilities, unless fitting into certain pant size becomes an Olympic sport or a path to empowerment (as of 2016, it is not).

A large portion of modern weightroom protocol squelches Frolic as we are taught to obey numbers and statistics. Play becomes work. Fun becomes obligation. We become less than human, not greater.

The last time most of us Westernized movers (and non-movers) had unregulated challenges against gravity, undocumented muscles creating force, movement free from clipboards or notebooks or formulas or tracking apps was at recess. Play is often synonymous with something essentially childish, and, like innocence and under-arm baldness, disappears as maturity set in. Grown-up. Adulthood. Words that seem to tow the line for seriousness. As mentioned earlier, play becomes hyper-competitive, war-like in many cases, or is eliminated entirely as we age. Frolic is long discarded.

The job of a trainer isn't simply to teach exercises. The duty of a coach isn't simply to yell motivation or start the clock ticking. No, the goal towards authentic strength is to cultivate Self-Awareness, Self-Reliance, and Self-Importance, which ultimately make you a much groovier member of your Tribe. Empowerment, as we've spewed many times, doesn't exist on a personal level unless it includes the Tribe.

Deep Recess

Remember 4th grade? Sitting at a desk for what seems like eternity, often under the frown of someone with some fairly unreal expectations of what you're supposed to deliver today... and for no observable reward?! Then, as if that's not enough, why not take some of that work home with you. Meanwhile you're being judged, graded, and picked apart by your peers, some of whom who call you 'friend.'

"Stressed out" might not be in the average 9-year-old's lexicon, but it ain't all fun and frolic. At this point in history you're at least a couple of years away from catching your best friend's brother rolling a joint in front of you, and the closest thing to hormonal demands on the heart, brain, and various other anatomical bits is hoping for that clandestine game of truth or dare to coerce Julie Vessel to kiss me on the cheek.

Oops.... did I switch tenses there? I wonder what happened to Julie. My cheek was never quite the same.

Not a lot of complaints about lower back pain or tension headaches though. Can we adults blame our current obsession with achy bits and joint creeks on age? Heck no, or at least not entirely. Age is simply the length of time we've had to make decisions, and if our choices were poor, that isn't the fault of chronology, no matter how much we shake a finger at the calendar.

Ironically, as we age, as the added responsibility of being grown up fills our cells with that elixir of destruction called stress, we also eliminate our stress-release valve.

Our 4th grade self had what could be argued as an equal amount of stress to our adult selves, if we create a relativity formula based on physical size, collected wisdom, and overall conscious coping options. Any waxing nostalgic we might do about the pre-teen years would be born from our yearning for those release valves that were available to us when we were hip high to a Grup[4].

We moved! And unless we had some sort of Bolshevik team coach, no one really told us HOW to move. We knew. We experimented. We explored. We played. Through movement of all varieties and intensities, we released tension. Judgment-free stress release. As movement maestro Jason C. Brown says (quoting a child) "Play is what I do when no one is telling me what to do."

We also learned.

Recess is strength, mobility, and creativity in action, in demand, in flux. Great word, 'flux.' Vaguely naughty sounding, yet not. Flux even played a role in the greatest invention of the 20th century: The time-traveling DeLorean.

Playfulness ranks high on the things-that-help-us-NOT-breakdown-through-aging list. Holding onto your youth, or embracing it after a period of not speaking to it is pretty similar to time travel. Recess: our own flux capacitor.

Oh wait, I hear that gossamer vibration of some young strength geek in the back shaking his head. He's thinking that, at 22 years of age, he's got decades before he has to worry about any of this. He can lift, screw, and fight with the best of them now, and it's all serious business. To him considering training as recess, movement as play, is anti-cool. He's a grown up now... no need for childishness. Just like mobility is yoga crap

---

[4] A slightly tricky Trekkie reference. Did you get it?

for "chicks and old people."

Up until his first injury. Might be when he's 23, might be when he's 43, but not understanding how the body truly wants to participate in the world will create a physical mutiny at some point.

A switch is flipped, sometime in our lives, where movement turns from joy to obligation, from recess to a workout. Movement, which was the territory of the body, switches to the territory of the brain. The bummer is that movement then switches from being a tension release valve to being just another stress. It becomes a time, a place, a schedule, a routine, a class, an exercise.

This might be an archaic reference reserved for those of us who grew up pre-internet. Can you remember the age in which you stopped going to your friend's house to ask them to come out and play? It was because you were a year or two into double digits, well on your way to adulthood. So you didn't do such childish things anymore. It was time to either stop moving or play a sport, and that was the beginning of the end.

What if we brought back movement as being a celebration of motion, being able to let the body do, learn and be? Here's the good news... if our brains have been successful wrapping themselves around the structured adult world of the modern workout, fear not! Successful play is served best from a foundation of structure. We can train for recess. In fact, the categorical protocols from all the years, studies, and bodies that have created the shifting world of training science can still play a role in play. As can our favorite tools.

Our over-the-pond buddy Rannoch Donald recently commented on the beauty of true and playful movement being the product of consistent practice. "We can train to play... but with play as our training!" A body wants the effort of conquering obstacles to achieve higher levels of ability. The challenges pay off in many ways. The body wants the beauty of the challenge and overcoming it, not just the outcome. I believe that's what we call strength.

Boy, does the industry offer it up in such an unappealing way, or at least I'm guessing our bodies think so.

9. Age: Pulling the Foot From the Grave to the Squat Cage

I'm...in disagreement about the...assertion – and the common belief – that diseases such as diabetes and cancer are due to aging and not simple lifestyle factors. These aren't diseases of aging, they're diseases of bullshit. We have this deeply ingrained belief, it seems, that aging inherently comes with disease and we're all just...well...screwed. Watch drug commercials and it would seem that once we hit 55, all that's left to do is retire, bicker about leftovers with the old ball and chain, and apparently settle in for a few decades of drugs, walkers, pee bags and pain prescriptions. But aging doesn't have to mean – and shouldn't mean – wrinkles, broken hips, weakness, and disease. Far from it. There's no reason you can't be as lean, strong, and energetic at 50, 60, 70, and even 80 as you were at 25. The key is not a drug, but a healthy, preventive lifestyle.
— Mark Sisson's Daily Apple Blog

Using age as an excuse is simply pointing the finger at the calendar rather than accepting the blame that you've gone a long time making poor decisions. I'm more than halfway to 90 as I write this, and my chronological journey brings a host of observations. No longer do I just have concern for friends and family that are in higher age classes. Now my concern is traveling the other direction. Who are you kids and why are you so decrepit?

You, in the skinny tapered jeans and those giant sunglasses that give you that cop-in-a-70s-porno look. Kudos for riding your fixed gear bike around town, but must you be smoking while you're doing it? Your posture is a chiropractor's dream, since, if you had any money, it could put his kids through culinary school (twice) with all the work it needs.

I've been out of college longer than you've been out of diapers. What choices are you making that your health should be so poor?

Why the rant? Huzzah, I say, to the trend of sagacity bringing people to better decisions. Although age is often the whipping boy, being blamed for any collection of ills, it is also with the wisdom that age brings that many are discovering the beauties of movement and strength later in life. Within BodyTribe walls hard work is expected, whether you're 20 or 200, and it is this rare equality that inspires me. We have a unique population where a good majority of our chronologically progressed tribe can kick the asses of the younger tribe members. This juxtaposition of tradition is almost comical to realize, since most eyes here don't see age and just see challenging play. This trend wasn't obvious until I actually considered the ages of our members. That makes me smile.

What if this role reversal of ability spread like a ripe avocado over the rest of the neighborhood? In my Utopian scenario, better choices are made as a body progresses chronologically. This dream gives me hope, for maybe this is the inspiration that changes a young mind to make better decisions at some point, after seeing a bunch of older bad-asses living fuller lives.

The older folks (like me) have always bitched about the younger ones (say, me in 1986). I'm now what I used to laugh at as a kid. "Shut up, old man," the 1986 Me would say to the current me. No, not really, I was too polite, but I'd be thinking it. Well, the current me could mop the floor with the 1986 me, and I'm planning on the 2026 me being able to do the same with the 2006 me. Nothing wrong with a little long term planning, eh?

Oh, if only I knew that then. As Oscar Wilde wrote, "I'm not young enough to know everything." Somehow that's appropriate.

Movement is good, but sometimes 'training' isn't. The brain invented training. The brain conceived the workout. The brain created this thing called exercise, and all the various categories it goes by (and all the various clichés it thrives on). The body has no idea what these things are. It just wants to move. In movement, the body knows better than the brain. Are we listening?

August, as my birthday month, has traditionally also been my competition season, as in the last 13 or so years I've decided to take gravity to the mat and enter some weightlifting or powerlifting or strongman meets to celebrate the new signifier in our human dance of chronology. Every year I strive for another kilo or two on the bar, and so far, I've been successful.

Now this flies in the face of our accepted idea of aging, which seems to promote a 'slow down and die already' concept of accruing more years in the calendar bank. This mistaken cultural standard begins with our culture's craving for peaking in our 20s, having our entire possible athletic prowess out of the way by the time we pass the quarter century mark. Our sports-centric, win-at-all-costs 'play' system desires our warriors to be their best before they've even experienced much of what the world offers. Too many stories have crossed my ears that began with "in college I..."

Then the downhill ride begins... and is supposed to continue in momentum for the next 40-80 years. At this point I should have at least 20 years of declining shimmer. Decay and rust should already have quite a hold on my joints, and atrophy is the only acceptable outcome for these ancient muscles.

These are the rules, so I am told regularly with a vehemence that is almost holy. Perhaps there is one thing we tend to forget a bit too easily...

Humans have so many possibilities at movement that we can spend our entire lives learning something new every single day, therefore never 'peaking.' Feel free to pick something to groove on for a while, but remember about the many options that could tickle our curiosity for the rest of our active, curious lives. We never need to Peak as a human unit. We never need to stare at an upcoming chunk of years as a perpetual rot of the system. In fact, that's kind of sick. We're the only mammals that limit ourselves like that. My 13-year-old cat is well past middle age, yet no one told him he's supposed to retire from being a moving, exploring creature. Aging is a mind game far before it is physical, and all other animals seem to know this except us. Infinite wisdom be damned.

Adding a kilo here and there (this year a snatch PR and a log clean and press PR) allows me to keep my chops sharp (an almost archaic turn of phrase these days). But the Olympic and strongman lifts are simply part of the foundation of my movement skills. If you know a thing or two about my programming (which you might after a few more chapters), they are simply catalysts for other skill training, allowing me to have some power and umph to put towards, well, anything I want. Remember... unlimited possibilities.

Did you know I suck at swimming? I mentioned my semi-fatal samba with H_2O on my blog, and since that experience, water and I have had a passionate, but strained, relationship (a common theme in my life). Water and I are far from strangers, as I've been participating in its pleasures forever, from snorkeling to cliff diving. These can all be deceptions, faked competency in the water. They require little swimming ability. Really. My comfort level in the drink is limited to things that require either unlimited floating (snorkeling) or a quick in-and-out (diving). Covering distance with any speed has led to some interesting scenarios, usually soul-crushing panic attacks only witnessed by a few unlucky folks. Last year I barely made it out to an island in the river and back without finding, and then changing, religions several times, and in the words of Justin Sullivan[5], praying to any god that would come.

This year I've been to the island several times. I've been swimming daily, mostly using the flaying breaststroke technique. I look like a drunk, legless moose trying to paddle with wings, but where I am not yet perfecting technique, I am overcoming fear. I am calm in the water. Still not great for distance, but better. This exploration was my biggest movement gift to myself this year, and I'm far from peaking, and even farther from declining.

Here's a lesson. Our training takes less work, if directed properly, to continue steady progress than you might think. If tomorrow means better than today, striving for huge leaps and bounds sets you up for a mountain that will be too tall to climb eventually. Sure, I preach Better trumps More, and it gets trumpeted all over social media when I mention it, but it surprises me at how few apply the idea.

Training is the organization of movement into a system for progress. This structure is where brain and body can learn from each other to create the best path. Brain listens to body's wants and needs, and then uses its calculating intelligence to create a path of physical education. Learning through moving, learning while moving, and moving to learn. This dialog is also why a 'program' of randomization makes little sense in a grand scheme of things.

---

[5] Singer/songwriter for New Model Army, who once personally replied to an email, and granted me permission to use a song of his for a video project of mine. For free. This means I've bought all their albums, and you should to.

Physical education. It's not your high school PE class.

Physical education is also why training and movement are not synonymous. At 46 years old, I can impress party goers with a few movement tricks, and can compete on a semi-competent level in various forms of strength athletics. I'm still getting better at these things every year, adding more tricks to my palette and more pounds on the bar. I can play harder now than I could 10, 15 or 20 years ago. Not because I'm a super amazing athlete. Far from it. In fact, being a skinny-ass bookworm musician in my early 20s, sort of an anti-athlete, helped me avoid planned obsolescence of my physical abilities. I didn't peak young and am making a conscious effort to avoid it now.

None of this means 'do not progress.' I think we've made a case for progression and peaking being two different things.

We're a smart bunch. Why do we either peak young or have to re-introduce movement back into our lives after avoiding it for many years since we were children? How about a middle ground, where we continue to embrace child-like play, that curious, exploratory passion for movement, into the years where we're told to chose between two movement options: either play sports (oh, and win, win, win), or quit being childish and therefore stop moving entirely?

Go ahead, talk among yourselves. What would a good middle ground be? How do we promote movement as a lifetime of progress, creativity, and education?

Let's overturn the current construct of movement-as-exercise. The embodied athlete knows that the journey trumps the outcome, that the big picture means learning from the small pictures. If we're listening to the body, then we don't have to win the workout.

Move more than train, play more that exercise. 'Let the body' far more than 'make the body.' In my roughly 11 years of competitive weightlifting (16 years powerlifting), I've upped my total the sum of what the specialized youngin's will get in a year. More importantly, I've racked up a handful of other groovy skills that enable me to enjoy movement beyond the gym. That total means little without the transfer to real life. I don't live for the gym; I live beyond it. Training is purposeful, intense movement to allow an even greater world of purposeful movement, even if the purpose is simply just to frickin' MOVE!

Strength athletics are simply a small part of my potential. Not my net worth. Competition is a benchmark of my journey, not the end result.

My child self is made better as an adult through training. With a tad of grown-up wisdom (do better, not more), it isn't a challenge to progress every year while engaging longevity, sans the danger of pushing extremes I don't have to. Don't get me wrong. I play on the edge during training and competition, just not with reckless abandon or unnecessary volume.

Think of this. If, at 46, I can add pounds to my bar or skills to my body with far less volume than kids in their 20's... why are they working so much? They're often doing 2 or 3 times the workload without 2 or 3 times the progress. Every workshop I teach is full of folks my junior who could out workout me. But I could out play them. My skill chunks are always increasing, while their volume is simply making them workout masters. Funny enough, with my limited time in the gym, I can still usually hold my own with their workouts as well.

But being an athlete isn't defined by time in the gym. If you can do less in the gym for more in life, shouldn't you? Trust me... you can.

10. Routine vs. Ritual

Character can now be communicated to a prospective client or new employer by the relative fitness of one's body. A lean, hardened body suggests discipline, control and personal responsibility. Great stamina suggests dedication. The qualities that a businessman admired - commitment, steadfastness and forbearance - are just as important today as they were a century ago. But now they are communicated differently. They are expressed through one's physique. The interpretation of character is now a completely visual process.

- Ronald Dworkin, <u>The Rise of the Imperial Self</u>

True or false? Not the statement itself. Dworkin is dead on in how judgment is made. But is it true about the actual judgment? Does a fit looking body translate to dedication or steadfastness?

If there is one thing anyone steeped in this Fitness Industrial Complex understands 100% is that what one looks like and what one actually is are not synonymous. Dworkin's not wrong about the perception, but the perception itself might be inaccurate. The modern fitness industrial light and magic show is the perpetuation of that perception to sell product without there being, in many (perhaps even most) cases, an actual correlation between a fit-looking body and real capability.

Nowhere in any substantial definition of fitness do the words "look better," "ripped abs," or "toned and defined" appear, yet these aesthetic quests make up for probably 90% of the Average Gym Members (AGMs) in the world. Since the premise of Dworkin's statement above is true (and the fitness industry is so happy it is), then many folks want to appear powerful (and the fitness industry will gleefully sell that to you). Judging a book by the cover, perhaps, but it's the quickest estimation of character we have. This prejudice may not be fair, but what else do you have to go on in the first few seconds of meeting someone?

Well, although the premise may be accurate, it shows a gross inaccuracy of character judgment. What may be initially perceived as dedication and forbearance may simply be narcissism or shallowness. Strength of character may correlate with strength of joints, muscle, spine and spirit, but rarely with just how pretty those muscles look.

These days it is easy to look the part without actually being the part.

The age-old correlation between aesthetic appeal and practical achievement is no longer entirely accurate (used to be, though), but the butt-whuppin' drive it takes to conquer our fitness demons is the same piss and vinegar we need for all other obstacles in life. Though Dworkin discusses simple appearance and how it relates to impressions, that belief exists because it's understood that by attaining a higher awareness of oneself through the mediums of intense movement and strength, the impressions of power, control and dedication won't be superficial. When we witness high levels of power and fitness in the gym (or out), we witness people who don't doubt their ability and set no limits on what they are capable of. That dedication often correlates with other areas of their life (hopefully). Unfortunately, people believe that looking the part equates to being the part. Common gym experience will belay time and time again how untrue that is.

Who's to blame for the emphasis on outer appearances? No one and everyone. "Blame" isn't exactly the right word. Our bodies process information quickly through the senses, sight usually being the first. Proper insight into someone takes more time and effort to incorporate deeper judgmental skills, to assess the worth of someone through achievement, ability, personality, etc., so our initial visual judgment holds until our minds process more information as we receive it. Since our initial perception is sensory based, it's a direct link to all our other sensory judgments, like physical attraction, which can easily override the brain's ability to create a fairer opinion based on more intrinsic and internal qualities. In other words, we can overlook a lot of personality flaws in physically beautiful people. Hence, the one night stand, or the long term, tumultuous relationship. Usually both are completely physically based, sometimes despite efforts to try to like or accept qualities about the other person that actually are quite annoying or downright disagreeable. It's easier (not better) for passion to exist from physical attraction – kickin' bod, nice smell, seductive smile - than from more profound attractions, like wisdom, common dreams and ideas, sense of humor. Our ubiquitous media is the largest exploiter of this. Therefore relationships and desires are created in greater numbers from the physical world, though they're often fickle, short lived, and erroneous. The strongest relationships, though, might begin with the physical, but then incorporate the spirit.

Our strongest pinnacles of culture, be it artistic (musicians, painters, writers) or cognitive activists (philosophers, religious idealists, politicians), have become attractive to us through a deeper, more powerful lust - the lust of the mind and spirit. After initially hitting our senses, we found something inside of us that embraced them, which replied back to our senses to ask for more. Our senses then were a means to an end, not the final decision, with the ultimate choice being a fulfilling internal, and eternal, one.

The tools needed for a true fitness lifestyle - dedication, focus and intensity - can be applied to all aspects of life, making any of us an even yummier part to our tribes through more than just an appealing flesh packet. This outcome is a definition of fitness: becoming better at life through movement. By improving the connection between body and mind we will make ourselves more useful, more inspiring, more "attractive" than just a pretty little flesh packet.

Incorporating the Spirit

"Spirit" often has religious or New-age connotations relating to foo-foo guru-ism or far-out fanaticism. Spirit, though, may be simply thought of as the untouchable, non-physical aspect of what drives our flesh packets. Fitness, then, is beyond physical. When our bodies, which house the ethereal essentials as well as the solid vitals, transcend the menial task of just holding everything together (in other words, when your body is fully alive) only then does the wall between flesh and spirit lower. Intensity, the quasi-tangible prerequisite for accomplishment, helps bridge the gap between body and soul. When we are pushed to the limits - intense pain, intense pleasure, intense terror, intense joy - concrete "goods" and "bads" fall on their foundations. Inner strength, sense of being, those obvious times when the spirit steps in to run the show, usually can be traced to a sensational intensity. We push our limits - physical, sexual, artistic, sensational - with a primal, subconscious desire to accomplish the incorporation of the spirit. Too often, though, the mind/body/spirit merger isn't completed, so steeped are we in just the physical, so content with our insecurities. We pull a "let's-just-be-friends" with our spirits, achieving only rare and brief samples of our potential in dreams, inspirations and epiphanies. We're too secure in our insecurities to accept the spirit through the threshold we often create for it.

Since intensity is a key to acknowledgment of the spirit, our workouts can make pretty strong bridges inward. This insight isn't to say that our training should be nothing but a self-actualizing quest. Heck, where's the fun in that? How about simply applying respect and appreciation for the art and science of movement? This gratitude will fulfill deeper needs than the constant struggle to look better. Let's face it. By following the three basics – train well, eat well, rest well – you're going to look better. It's a required by-product. When that focus dominates a workout, though, the accomplishment is rather shallow, a minor victory in your grand scheme.

Inspiration and celebration for life

We need basic functions and actions to provide ourselves with the ability to transcend basic functions and actions. We wake up, brush our teeth, pretty-up ourselves, dress, and eat before we attack the greater tasks of creating, accomplishing, and providing. Though your protocol might not match the exact pattern above, we all have routines to move us through the day so we can focus and function better on more important tasks. Routines are thoughtless actions that meet basal requirements. Routines do not offer inspiration or purpose beyond our most simple needs. Routines, albeit necessary, are droll. Plain and simple.

Fitness goals are more often vague hopes than thought-out plans. Most folks in the gym "will know when they get there," which is to say they don't have measured steps and progressions that can be manipulated to ensure progress. Fitness goals are rarely about life enhancement (unfortunately) and have more to do with simple, often erroneous or obsessive, aesthetic goals (which actually negates them having anything to do with "fitness").

Movement, especially in extreme forms, is an open spectacle, an individual parade for existence. The ability to overcome very real and physical obstacles, be it in the form of several hundred pounds lifted off your body or conquering new terrain on a cardiovascular journey, should never be a routine. Let's not take motion for granted.

When asked "how do we live spiritually?' Joseph Campbell replied, "In ancient times, that was what ritual was for. A ritual can be defined as the enactment of a myth. By participating in a ritual, you are actually experiencing a mythological life. And it's out of this participation that one can learn to live spiritually"

When conscious thought or meaning is applied to a movement or task to invoke a greater good, then it is a ritual. When considering what Dworkin wrote, instead of gaining the appearance of power and discipline, why not actually *be* powerful and disciplined?

> "People create images of themselves in the world and guide their action according to such images. The images are not only myths that capture the meaning of past experiences but lead to anticipation of future events." - N. Fredman and R. Sherwood, Handbook of Structured Techniques in Marriage and Family Therapy

The meaning of myth in ritual is not folklore, or storyteller's fantasy, but the correlating metaphoric representation of strong, and quite real emotion, aspect, or quality in life. With ritual within a workout, a lift cannot only be a literal display of power, but also representative of power in other aspects of life, a very real myth of power. Much of the fitness literature out there makes wonderful, if not oblique, claims of self-empowerment, stress relief, or ability to deal with stress better, esteem building, and the overcoming of many non-physical obstacles. These aren't, unfortunately, just automatic byproducts of fitness. Unless some cognitive effort is made not to take physical ability for granted, these potential qualities are wasted. Obligatory fitness, which is fitness under duress of guilt, usually stemming from erroneous pressures of physical ideals, will not meet any of the above claims. Obligatory fitness makes up for that giant dessert from last night, or a weekend of binging. It is fitness without ritual, fitness without passion. It yields little true gain and satisfies daily guilt, not any actual goal.

Okay, so now what?

> "To derive power from a ritual it must, in some way, stand apart from our ordinary lives. It is not uncommon for us to have so much of our energy and attention directed towards our daily routines and our goals that our focus becomes narrowed. We may even have become preoccupied with our doubts, our fears, or our pain. These things can isolate us. We may lose connection with the rhythm in our lives and the passage that we share as human beings on the planet. This is what the existential philosopher Martin Heidegger called a state of 'forgetfulness of being.'" - Renee Beck and Sydney Metrick, The Art of Ritual

A common and easy way to dwell in the "forgetfulness of being" is to live in routine. Now routines can have an acceptable, if not required, place in survival as mentioned earlier. But a routine in itself is not progress, nor does it create progress. Routine is simply the foundation from which inspiration might have a spring board. By being self-aware, and "conscious of being the creative composer of one's own life" (Beck), we achieve the condition of "mindfulness of being." We can take a little responsibility, using our workout as one of many possible vehicles, and choose to be aware of our movements and action, maybe even using a little metaphor or fantasy to shift the focus from the micro process (sets, reps, mechanics) and view its place in the macro process (being better at life). If we view our workouts as ceremonies of intensity and commitment and apply them to an organized set of cyclic goals, from baby steps to the grand scheme o' things, the workout can become a ritual, not just a routine.

Even famed malignant Englishman Aleister Crowley wrote "magick is the art and science of making change occur according to will." If our true will is simply droppin' some fat to satisfy a scale, then we should be damned to a life of obligatory fitness. If our workouts are rituals of the celebration of movement, ability, and therefore life, we're pretty magickal.

11. Transformation

Purpose and transformation are life partners. One finishes the other's sentences. When their eyes met for the first time, they both breathed, "you complete me." One can't quit the other. Unless you're perfect in every way (therefore not needing transformation), your time steeped in that purposeful recess of training is simply the consecration of their union.

Well, sorta. Purpose is actually one third of the recipe. But let's not jump too far ahead.

The Recipe for Transformation
   1) Intensity
   2) Consistency
   3) Purpose

That's it. That's the alchemy for your transformation. Here's how it works.

Intensity ignites the potential for transformation, as we've mentioned in Ritual vs Routine. It is the spark for change. It's also the focus of the next chunk of this book.

Consistency is simply repeating this ignition until it's a fire. It perpetuates the change.

Purpose defines the change! This is perhaps the biggest theme of this tome. Not all transformation is good. Random or aimless encounters with intensity have no direction, and therefore the outcome might, well, suck. Even well-intentioned attempts at transformation can be badly programmed, steering the intensity through a series of poor choices, which, as we'll chat more about, reduce our options and limit our freedom.

We've waxed ad nauseum about purpose throughout these pages, so what needs some serious crime scene investigation is the concept of intensity. We've already let the ink dry on it's importance to our ritual. What the heck does it mean?

Do Better: The Story of Intensity

Through the omnipresent lens of social media, I'm witness to many prescribed workouts by many trainers and gyms across the world. A great deal of them fall into a theme of do-more-faster, with various workouts prescribing hundreds of reps. One recent example was a workout of 200 air squats/100 KB swings/50 pushups/50 box jumps[6], then repeat for half of everything, for a grand total of 600 reps. That's a lot. Yet that's becoming standard programming. Is there a point? Later we'll also ask the question: Why would such programmed redundancy be at all appealing to the huge chunk of the population we need to be trying to get moving? Why has movement become regulated, and often celebrated, repetition?

Only a few bits of wisdom will seep through my old, calloused cranium, but a big lesson that has lodged itself in that pink orb between my ears is that quality trumps everything. Why do my athletes improve? They work on doing things better. Since our big journey is the path towards holistic usefulness, then it may behoove us to place a great deal of importance on the carry-over from workout to real life. Hence it is crucial to recognize that quality of life often has a direct

---

[6] Don't worry if you're unfamiliar with any of these movements. That's not the point.

correlation with the quality of your training... but less so directly with the quantity.

With that formula for transformation, the magic goop that puts glitter on our unicorn horn is Intensity. When we repeat it (Consistency) and give it direction (Purpose), we're changed. Simple. Depending on that purpose, we might be one step closer to actually being useful.

This diatribe ain't new gospel from my pulpit. In fact the premise of BodyTribe is the quest for intensity as a game, and life, changer. Strength is ability. Physically, it's the ability to overcome obstacles. Metaphysically... well, basically the same thing. Face a challenge and deal with it. As with mastery of anything, we practice it. Our physical training is simply creating challenges and then slapping them around to make them our bitch. Or at least attempting to.

Therein lies a dilemma. Our limited time on this cosmic spinning glitter orb is already rife with challenges. Why would anyone want to create more challenges? Why would we want to purposely put real physical obstacles in our own way, simply to go over them, under them, or move them?

Because it is a skill, this obstacle crushing. To improve our skills, we should practice. Frankly, in our quest for humanness, these challenges are what make things interesting. Even fun.

The good news is that we can have a blast doing it. The outcome, says those around us, is, as we mentioned earlier, an increase in our **mate-able worth**. Oh, and the real big news? There will be ass kicking in the future. Your tribe gains a superhero, if you choose to use your powers for good (and you will... that's why I like you).

Why is volume not always the answer? Isn't Volume intense? Hold on, my friends, we'll be there soon. Sure, all transformation comes from challenge, but not all challenge creates transformation. We call this the classic Coaches Fallacy.

First, what is Intensity?

Don't Google this one. It won't quite solve the riddle. I see the strength athletes with their hands up. Calling on one of them would get me an answer about percentage of 1RM. Intensity for them is the all-out kaboom of a max effort lift.

The metcon junkies are going to counter this with a power output proposition. The yoga contingent will pitch a case for focus and awareness.

And yes, someone will make a case for volume. Doing a lot of something feels awfully intense, right?

You are all right, but it's a math question, and none of you showed your work. Well, metaphysical math, but Intensity is a formula nonetheless.

Intensity = investment X challenge

That's right. Intensity is the amount of investment times the level of challenge. Simple, right?

Now we're masters at busy-ness, which is a bunch of investment in unchallenging things. On the other hand, many of us have strangleholds on walking away from giant challenges, maybe after a half-ass effort, what I call the At Least I Tried Syndrome. Those, obviously, fail at being transformative. According to our formula, not much intensity.

The examples of intensity given earlier, though – 1RM, focus, metabolic meltdown – all plug into our equation with a net sum of a **high intensity quotient**. So yes. Intensity can come from volume. High numbers represent a big challenge, and if met with high investment, your intensity formula will definitely ring in the red zone.

Beware. Not all intensity is the same.

Can intensity be abusive? Heck yes. Its transformative powers can turn metal into gold or shit into a bigger pile of shit. I've oft quoted the legendary Tommy Kono as saying **practice makes permanent.** If you're finding your intensity through practicing a volume fest of crap, guess what you're making permanent?

12. Building and Breaking the Machine

We're organic machines. We come out of the factory (so to speak) unfinished, but with a ton of built-in software and potential. We differ from manufactured machines in that we create ourselves, and, of course, we're hylomorphically connected to the software that accompanies the hardware.

Intensity can turn us into super high performance vehicles for an equally amazing physical and metaphysical collection of components and programming. We can't forget, though, that we share something very important with manufactured machines...

Abuse it and lose it.

A manufactured machine is ready for its purpose once it leaves the factory floor. Rev that sucker up and expect horsepower. That's its reason for existing, and modern technology lets us create it so it can do its thang fresh out of the box.

You are not that machine. Our organic nature means you're a machine that builds itself. If we skip this building process, we will break. However, we have something in common with the manufactured machine: that little characteristic of a flaw perpetuating itself. If a machine begets a minor change in its structure that even ever so slightly changes the original plan of its movement, the machine will wear down and you can plan on big problems eventually. In other words, anything that changes the correct process of the machine, no matter how small, will make a big mess at some point.

As an organic appliance, not only might your physical systems not yet be up for huge horsepower tasks, you might not even have the benefit of being programed with the right idea of what movement should be, especially if the workload demand is high. High rep-for-speed training, especially for a beginner who never learns anything different, can easily skip the steps of embodiment.

For anyone, any *body*, doing MORE may actually shut down the communication between mind and body. It becomes trauma control time, and the mind switches to 'just get through this anyway possible,' which are never buy-words for quality. The body, or mind, doesn't learn the movements. The dialog has ended and the workout has actually become a greater stress on the body than previously existed.

Let's state trauma to the hylomorphic machine in a more dramatic, but accurate, fashion: The modern protocol of Do More Faster can actually create a trauma survival response. Sure, to the uninformed, this might sound like a desired outcome, and they'll read this as 'training like that helps survive through trauma.' Wrong. Dead wrong. That type of training *becomes* the trauma. And that, as any trauma survivor will tell you, is *never* a desired situation to be in. It is DISembodiment, a shut down between mind and body. This becomes an extreme version of the Slave Driver archetype, where the mind is entered into a battle for survival, and forcing the body to get through the process is not actually considered a win. Hormonally, emotionally, and at levels of the psyche and nervous system your conscious self may not be privy to, purposely putting yourself through that dysfunctional relationship has ramifications that are hugely detrimental to multiple layers of your being.

Nothing about a self-perpetuated trauma cycle creates an authentic relationship with your body. Quite the contrary. If you're a fitness professional, spend some time working with trauma survivors to understand how purposeful abuse, in this case through exercise, even if the intentions are good(ish), can create a lifetime of problems.

Stress is a big part of fitness training, and is actually part of the challenge/empowerment journey. But when we skip mastery of movement, skip embodiment, skip intensity through listening to your body, and go straight for the trauma, we've replaced adaptation and achievement with abuse.

Plus, on a purely physical level, the chances of your biological packaging acquiring a misfire in its performance is way beyond that of a manufactured machine... heck, it's almost mandatory. The consequences are a bit more dire. Our machines, pretty amazing regardless, need programming and practice to be the best machines they can be. Remember that next time you feel like attempting a high rep-for-speed workout. Do you truly know the movements? Are you built and programmed for it yet? Most importantly, is there a good reason for doing it?

In other words, Intensity as abuse does create change. *It breaks the machine.*

Our training should be full of many malleable factors to physically create intensity within a workout... speed, movement selection, position, presence, time, duration, distance, load and, of course, volume (and the metaphysical list of options is spread throughout this book). When I see 50+ reps of a movement within a combo or WOD, it usually indicates that volume was the *only* factor changed to increase intensity, and when that is the basis of a program, it's a glaring rookie move.

There are often way better choices. A rep is not just a rep, so adding more of them might often be the last thing to consider. There are too many effective ways to eek the most out of the rep(s) before choosing to do more of them, whatever the goal. If you can do 50 reps, that's your body saying okay, we got this, now let's change the gosh-darn challenge already. Heck it was probably saying that at rep 10 or 20.

Using the original WOD mentioned at the beginning, there are many far more important things I'd want to know about my athletes before I want to know if they can do a total of 300 air squats. High volume through repetition should be quite low on the Good Coaching priority list.

Keep in mind; the Authentic Athlete strives for usefulness. Coaching that athlete means understanding Purpose. Intensity is directed by that purpose.

Intensity is your best friend and most brutal mentor. Yup, sometimes intensity looks like a heavy, intimidating object, other times a grueling collection of tasks. On the other side of the coin we have stillness, reflection, play, or understanding, as concepts with very intense properties. There is a good chance they'd be greater tools in the transformation arsenal than simply volume.

Yes, we'll explore some options throughout this book.

13. Create a More Complete Program
(Intensity Through Planning)

Strength geeks have dwelled in caves, basements, and garages for decades, doing stuff that the modern Fitness Industrial Complex pretends doesn't exist. The raw goop of blood, sweat, tears, and the occasional remix of lunch might be the proven recipe for a better you and me, but it's a tough sell, so the corporate fitness world had to use shiny things and catchy words to make their millions, uh, billions, off of insecurities and fears. **The foundation of our** entire fitness industrial complex was originally built around this concept, if you'll remember:

You are ugly. We can help.

Therefore hard work was out. Gadgets, gizmos, and apparel were in. People bought it. They ran in place, cycled in place, sat on benches and lay on the ground to 'exercise,' hoping that someday the mirror and the scale were going to tell them they didn't suck so badly.

Meanwhile, those caves, basements, and garages were cranking out people who could DO things and prided themselves on accomplishments beyond the mirror and scale. What the fitness industry had a hard time avoiding was that these folks usually looked pretty damn good, since that is the required outcome of hard work and eating right. You look strong because you ARE strong.

Strong is, in a word, hawt!

That was still hard to sell. So real strength and fitness remained underground for many years. We dubbed this brand of heavy playtime as the Physical SubCulture. It was a small handful of strength and movement freaks, and an even smaller number of gyms, around the world, creating strength and ability in the tradition of the physical culture movement of a century ago, when people who cared about themselves worked hard, played hard, and experimented with their limitations. They'd also write groovy prose like this:

> *Action is life, power, success. Inaction is failure, impotence, death. Proper action is the basis of all physical, mental, and moral progress.* – David P Butler, 1868

Over the last decade or so, the previously unaware general public has been slowly introduced to some of these concepts and tools, despite the best efforts of the Fitness Industrial Complex working even harder at promoting uneducated marshmallow workouts or aesthetically driven bodybuilder protocols... stuff that is easy to teach, sell and market, but doesn't actually make for a capable human.

Over time the modern physical culture movement has been inching its way out of the 'subculture' status as the curious and hungry masses began actually wondering if they were, all this time, being duped by a bullshit industry. The bravest among them began embracing movement and strength traditions that had lived so quietly in the shadows for so long, and programs, techniques, and philosophies about strength, ability and maybe even a little embodiment, began to find new eyes, ears, muscles and minds.

This development has been both good and bad.

Folks are now a bit less hesitant to at least shake hands with these odd and old ways of moving. Some programs and philosophies, such as ours at BodyTribe, are being embraced by a fitness world ready to accept that real movement and strength, not the packaged fitness that's been sold for so long, could be what their personal journeys are supposed to be. Not bad, right?

Well, with new blood often comes diluted understanding. The new breed of teachers and coaches often haven't the depth of thought, or spent the time under the bar, or time at the master's feet, needed to truly pass on the lessons and traditions that sometimes need a few lifetimes to appreciate. Anything resembling an apprentice process has become a 2-day certification, and now there are too many folks teaching what they, the teachers, barely comprehend. The insta-expert process is the new fad amongst the popularizing of the once underground Physical SubCulture. Despite the growing trend of barbells and this pseudo-physical culture that is spreading, most of the new breed of fitness professionals are still in proverbial diapers when it comes to introducing force to the body in strange and intense ways. Passion alone doesn't create a trainer or coach, nor does a few initials after your name. As mentioned earlier, we're a tad too quick handing out the label of "coach" these days.

Not only are many of the coaches new to applying movement to other bodies, they're also painfully unaware of the many, *many* possible better options for movement, technique and even program design (all different paths to Intensity) that might be out there. The narrow focus of the cults of programming approach knowledge like getting a bachelor's degree in a particular subject without even realizing there were other majors, higher levels of degrees, or even other colleges.

But wait, there's more. When we have a big ol' crush on something, but don't quite comprehend its true depth, we must label and categorize it. Then we have some control over it, plus we can then sell it. Movement became exercise and exercise became cardio/resistance training/flexibility training. Then the deeper subculture of real strength started being the freshly poked bear, and new categories emerged, like flow/crossfit/mobility/animal/ primal/kettlebell/ powerlifting/weightlifting... and more.

Instead of pursuing movement as a passion, we need the hubris and labels to understand, and buy and sell, these new (or my favorite, "unconventional") concepts. This structuring, unfortunately, has led to more limits, not less. More boundaries instead of fewer. More excluding, rather than uniting.

For one big reason. The original message ("serving the ugly since forever") had to change. It became:

"What we're doing is better than what you're doing."

All of it misses the point. They're all simply ways of plugging in that Intensity formula. Unfortunately a tribe will often become a bit territorial about their idea (brand) of Intensity. They soon forget that Intensity has many faces.

But first, some history...

The year was 1995. Forrest Gump answered the question of what stupid was. Pam and Tommy did the same thing by tying an unfortunate knot (and the world watched as he steered a boat with his endowment). Jerry Garcia, grateful or not, died.

It was also the year that a new trend in fitness began to shape up, so to speak. New to the scene were these big, inflatable balls that brought fitness to a whole new level. So simple, yet so effective for developing this new rage called your core. The fit ball, or the Swiss ball, or the Resist-a-Ball™, this instant fitness classic was the TRX of the times. Showy, fun, but not really the best bang-for-the-buck. Although more circus act than powerhouse (just like the TRX... yeah, not a huge fan), the fit ball in the mid-90's was about to become the Next Big Thing.

It isn't without a slight bit of embarrassment that I admit to a little known fact. I was the first Resist-a-Ball certified trainer in California. But that isn't the actual story here. To acquire this cert, one of the 14 or so I collected in the early years when I thought such things mattered, I had a delightfully educating trip to the wonderful town of Carlsbad, CA, where I spent a weekend with some of the most entertaining, and in some cases, irritating, biomechanics geeks I'd yet to encounter at that point in my training life. Arguments such as the correct degree of shoulder joint angle to achieve the greatest rear deltoid recruitment (yeah... at a big, bouncy ball workshop) abounded, all with complete sincerity.

The favorite little bit of knowledge I walked away that weekend with was about the building that housed the workshop. A decent sized fitness studio that was home to Jazzercize HQ. Even 20 years ago, some of us had to ask if Jazzercise was still around, and apparently it was (is).

Quick bit o' facts from the interweb: "In 2009/2010 Jazzercise reported 96 Million in revenue. On the 2011 Entrepreneur Franchise 500 list, Jazzercise ranks as the #1 fitness franchise and #17 overall. In March 2009, MSNBC placed Jazzercise in their top 5 list of proven franchises that provide growth opportunity." I'm not about to research much more on its current business model, but all of this popularity was in full swing back in the mid 90's when I had my weekend education during my stint in Carlsbad. Back then I learned that every year the institution that is Jazzercise creates a routine that can be easily taught. That routine lasts the entire year, so Jazzercised travelers can visit a jazzercise studio anywhere and already know the steps. Last I heard, this model is still in place.

Let this prelude just be a little story not only about the length of time I've been in this industry, but also the lifespan and evolution of certain trends. An interesting irony: despite its almost 1 billion dollar industry chunk, I couldn't tell you where a local Jazzercise facility is. In my mind, they're more underground than Olympic lifting gyms, Crossfits, or kettlebell dens, of which I can point to almost a dozen within a couple of miles from me. If being unknown is the litmus for cool, who is hardcore now? Jazzercise... the hipsters of fitness.

Back to the point, which was that we're easily distracted

by big bouncy balls, or whatever The Next Big Thing happens to be. A trainer's history can often be judged by their outdated collection of gadgets. Months, if not years, might be wasted down rabbit holes of hoping that our trend of choice will be the game changer it was hyped up to be. Because of our fad-loving behavior, the constantly growing fitness industry is holding itself back from being an amazing, and world-changing, network. Currently there are limitless possibilities, but only occasional successes (you know who you are). This modern explosion of enthusiastic nouveau trainers will quite likely get as sidetracked as the generations before them. The Next Big Thing will replace the usable knowledge of movement, force development, and the human relation to both. Where does that leave the general public? Lacking. Sometimes practical ability is usurped by silly human tricks. Hindsight of my own history reminds me of this lament.

In other words, we're breeding a lot of empty trainers. This vacuum of depth doesn't bode well for non-trainers who simply want to move and be strong. They'll have to look beyond the industry for some real lessons.

Here's a recent example. At a giant fitness convention I met a pair of young women (drinking age would have to be proven) who were raving about their equally young coach, strutting behind them, and about how brilliant his workouts were. After hearing a bit about his ideas on programming, it was obvious that not only were these workouts a tad short of brilliant, but that none of them knew anything much different. Apparently rule number one of being a trainer (coach... so be it) is simple: An audience who doesn't know any better is easy to impress. Heck, that's the entire M.O. of the fitness industry. Be loud, be intense, be enthusiastic, and the general public, who doesn't know any better, will shout "revolutionary!" Enthusiasm, more so than actual quality, lends to the rise of any fitness trend, no matter how hard we try not to believe that. Personality, remember?

Here's the good news...

A lot of modern ideas aren't bad ones. Do some quality work using quality movements to create some quality intensity. Keep said quality high and you should have some quality results. That formula, on paper, is a good absence of bullshit. Simple. Basic. And, as is well understood in the iron game, simple is not synonymous with easy, so the workouts will be anything but.

But...

To create all this quality, you need a bit of lurnin', a bit of spirit, a bit of passion, and a good heaping of free thought. Like any art, craft, or skill, some serious study and application needs to happen before you load up another human being (or yourself) with some iron and make them move fast. The absence of this wisdom is why the current execution of the modern trends, certifications and programs falls short.

What can be done? Well, if you'd care to read on, I've jotted a few ideas here. Keep in mind this simple premise...

There is no talent in creating a hard workout. A good workout, on the other hand, requires a greater degree of understanding. Do you know the difference?

If Intensity is the spark for transformation, let's understand many ways to achieve it. We'll chat about it in the next few chapters.

14. Potential Versus Actual Strength
(Intensity Through Load)

What follows is a discussion on the proliferation of some modern misguided training programming. If your movement journey is relatively new, perhaps what follows will be a primer for what you will bare witness to soon. If you're a card-carrying, certified member of the current fitness industrial complex, this is familiar territory.

Matt Wichlinski, who has added WWE strength coach to his resume (which may be the 2nd or third coolest job in the world), and I were Skyping about strength one day (as such geeks do), and we quickly realized we had the exact same definition for Strength. If you've kept up with my blog over the decade+ it's been around (it began as a series of posts on a Yahoo group over 15 years ago), you might already be quick to shout out that strength = ABILITY!

In fact, trainers (coaches, whatever) tend to agree that training is our tool to get good at stuff. Ya know... building skills.

And yet...

The biggest skill folks seem to be building in the gym is the ability to workout. We have no guarantee that anything we do in the gym transfers to that big chunk of life beyond the gym. The correlation between the iron and the rest of our lives actually has be an important component of your programming. Yep, that's right. You have to program potential strength into actual strength. The observations from these cheap seats where my butt dwells are that there doesn't seem to be a lot of that.

All the pulls, ups, downs, pushes, snaps, boings, and kabooms we do in the gym are meant to create potential. Programming will decide the degree of usefulness, the amount of transfer, that potential has. Here's a quick example... The infamous burpee. As you've probably noticed, whether you're ankle- or ass-deep in this stuff, a burpee can be done as a floppy mess or it can be a well-tuned production between two major body alignments we call 'shapes.' Understanding and practicing the shape model, which we'll chat about a little later, will create an awareness, and a potential for embodiment, that has an easy transfer to other aspects of movement and athleticism, even if the numbers are small. The spasming worm style, on the other hand, has about as much potential for furthering other skills as learning to dance by watching John Hughes films. Adding more icky reps is, as mentioned many times before, practicing slop. Since practice makes permanent, where would that leave you?

It doesn't take a giant leap to see how your training might not actually help your ability to take a giant leap. Does an 800 pound squatter instantly have mad skills at the other foundations of movement? That squatter has probably taken his training *beyond* the point of usefulness, choosing instead to create potential in one thing: standing up with a heavy bar on his back. He now squats to get better at squatting, rather than using the squat to get better at anything else.

If strength is ability, he is actually fairly limited in his strength, whereas a 500 pound squatter who hasn't squandered his time on an all-squat diet, but instead uses that squat as simply a tool for building potential at other strengths/skills, could be considered less limited in his strength. If we sum up our potential as usefulness, then the 'weaker' squatter would have more potential, therefore being more useful. More skilled. More able. In other words, stronger.

Gasp

Let's continue this game.[7]

A common quest for the nouveau fitness culture is a little exercise aggressively named a muscle-up. A muscle-up is a basic ring skill, like kindergarten for gymnasts. Sure, pretty challenging for mere mortals, but considered an entry level gymnastics skill that is meant for one thing: To get up on something so you can then DO OTHER THINGS. It's the intro level to getting up on bars or rings, so you can then create a greater movement palette. Once you have the ability to do a few, if you're going to increase potential, ask yourself what's next? The answer is not DO MORE OF THEM FASTER! What potential would that be building? Once you have a handful under your belt, graduate. Move on. That's their purpose as a movement... to get you to the *beginning* of something. Turning the muscle-up into a high rep workout, or better yet, part of a sport, is like being a 8-year-old in preschool. You've mastered step one into the ground. You've made a sport of the warm up from another sport. You've sucked the potential right out of it by giving it more importance than it should have. What an interesting programming decision to make.

We could play this game all day. Box jumps seem to be trending right now, that workout staple of hopping up onto a little box, usually repeated for so many reps it looks like punishment rather than accomplishment.

A box jump is not as much a skill you need to build, as it is an outcome from other skills. Getting good at high rep box jumps doesn't make you particularly good at much else, while training other more potential-building skills will actually make you a competent box jumper. There was a viral video of Olympic weightlifters hopping up onto enormous stacks of

---

[7] What will be interesting is how the following section holds up under time, since exercise trends come and go. In 10 years, will the following references seem archaic? Probably.

bumper plates almost as tall as they are. Don't think for a minute they acquired their mad box jumps by practicing tons of box jumps. That skill is an outcome of their explosive training (Olympic lifting), not the actual task itself (box jumping).

In other words, you can build the very simple skill of hopping on a box by practicing bigger, more important skills. But those more important skills don't benefit much from constant box jumps.

I know, I know, you're using box jumps as a conditioning tool, as a movement to build the skill of fighting fatigue. Who cares if it, in itself, is a skill worth building?

Aren't there better choices? I bet you could find them, and your client's shins (and morale) would appreciate it.

I get it. A current big trend is to covet power output as a skill, the ability to do more stuff faster. It is, in fact, a pretty useful one. The point of power output, however, is to create a potential foundation of stamina to then be able to practice and improve *other skills*. It, in itself, isn't the key to potential. Power output is a support player to a bigger picture. It *is* a skill; it just isn't *the* skill. Creating entire programs based on doing more, faster, misses the entire point. In fact, they're backwards.

When we reduce the potential of other skills by creating high rep, low load, speedy versions of them in the name of power output, we're actually reducing the potential of our programming.

Power output is not technique practice or higher skill building. Now that power output, and its minion, 'workload,' have trumped maximum force/skill development as the ruler of the programing kingdom, our organic machines are falling victim to this backwards trend.

Backwards? Yup. Strength trickles down. Having a solid base of high levels of force development, in fact going towards the far end of the strength spectrum into what we call Maximum Force Development (MFD), what might be recognized as good ol' fashioned STRENGTH to conventional eyes, transfers greater to the Foundational Skills, and Big Picture Skill Chunks that we'll talk about later. That foundation is the solid ground we should build on, and bringing up our work capacity and power output is simply a tool to utilize our MFD better. Power output ("GPP", "Metcon", etc) is simply applying our ability to generate force on a broader scale. It also helps us sustain a larger training schedule to get towards those increases in max force, which is generally synonymous with mad skill development.

In other words, power output supports MFD. It is a helper in a cycle of generating greater force. It is not THE foundation of a program, but a tool to help support what should be the foundation, which is MFD. To generate maximum force properly, you might wanna work on technique. In fact MFD is interchangeable with Maximum Skill Development (MSD), since perfecting an important foundation skill requires, well, MFD (but that's more programming than we're going to discuss here).

An athlete with building potential in MFD/MSD will be able to train down the spectrum of strength into high rep workload training far easier than the opposite. You can make a quality strength athlete good at CrossFit or endurance feats faster than going the other direction.

Point being, program design is a big, fun-filled world beyond just doing a bunch of stuff as fast as possible, but so many of the trends in physical culture right now seem bent on more, faster. Not more, BETTER, which has been the fool-proof plan of the truly strong for centuries before hand. The body likes a good challenge. "Good" as in quality. Use volume only if the quality is maintained. Otherwise it's anti-fitness. Anti-skillful.

What follows includes some maths. It also includes talk about programming and training (despite my saying I wasn't going to talk much about programming) and exercise stuff that could quickly bore some of you, especially if your fitness journey is less of a profession, more of a passion. You may skip onward and not lose a beat, if you'd like to chat more about the deeper thought of moving. For you trainer/coach folks, though, this will hammer home some big truths. These big truths might not jive with the maths you've been basing your truths on. Y'all been warned.

The Myth of Power Output as The Ring That Binds Us All.

Power output is measured by work over time. Do a bunch fast. The more overall weight you can move quickly, the more Power you have. 100 cumulative pounds done in 1 minute is more 'powerful' than 90 pounds done in the same time, or even 190 pounds done in 2 minutes, for example, since the power output would only then be 95 pounds a minute.

Let's take a famous example. In the CrossFit world, she's called Fran, one of the famous CF challenges carrying a woman's name.

If you're not familiar with her, Fran is a workout consisting of the following: Squat presses[8] and pull ups (and, let's face it, for most these will be kip ups... using the entire body to pop the body up with more momentum than muscle). With a rep scheme of 21/15/9, as fast as you can.

Although the barbell is set at 95 pounds for men, let's round up the weight to 100 pounds, just to make this math easy. A decent Fran time is under 4 minutes, so 45 total reps at 100 pounds would be 4,500 pounds of work completed for that task. Qualifying the pull up is harder. Let's just use bodyweight of the person, in this case a 200 pound athlete, so 9000 pounds of pull up work. All done in 4 minutes, for this example.

---

[8] Despite them now often referred to as 'thrusters' I'm still calling them squat presses to avoid the ridiculous imagery of some dance move inspired by watching too much porn.

So, to sum up, example 1:

4,500 pounds of squat presses.

9,000 pounds of pull ups.

All done in 4 minutes.

What if we doubled the load of the thruster? Then we simply change the pull up by enforcing that they be strict. And we reduced the reps to 10/7/4. The maths:

4,100 pounds of squat presses.

4,100 pounds of pull ups.

Maybe they even went a little slower. In fact, we'll say the whole thing takes 5 minutes.

So far, by formula, the power output is considerably lower. But I dare you to argue that such a workout would be any less productive... if you could even pull it off.

Now let's double the load again for the squat presses. Yup, a 400-pound squat press. We'll add 100 pounds to the pull up by hanging a weight from our fictional character. This scenario isn't *that* far from reality. I've known at least a couple of folks who could probably pull this off at 200 pounds of bodyweight. Now let's reduce their reps way down to 5/3/2.

Total pounds of squat presses: 3,800

Total pounds of pullups: 3,000

Let's say it went slightly speedier, back to 4 minutes. That would still be a slow, much worse performance, according to the power output model.

Who would you want on your team? To save your family from a hurricane full of zombies and werewolves? Heck, to hang out with as a person? The person with the greatest potential here would be the final example, and if you see otherwise, remind me not to pick you for my dodgeball league.

See it this way: who can become the other the easiest? Person #3 can become Person #1 easily. But Person #1 has a heck of a lot of work to do to reach even Person #2's status, and never will by training with that low weight version of the power output model. So why would we put the majority of our training into a lower outcome of potential? Why would we train primarily like Person #1 if we see that Person #3 is more of an ideal of potential? Person #3 surely didn't get that way by following Person #1's programming.

This little comparison game of athletic make-believe above is simply an example of how our identity can be dogmatically tied up in just one quest for intensity, where we may not only hamstring ourselves physiologically, but philosophically as well. Think better, move better... and vice versa.

15. If It's Too Loud, You're Too Old… or Weak.
(Intensity Through Play)

I'm 46-ish years old (so far). According to some sacred wisdoms, I've had time to work on my jig, memorize my capitals, and conjugate my verbs. I've still got some centuries in me yet to sail the world, write the great American novel (or ebook), and perfect my long division, but all in good time. Slowing down is not an option. Sure it takes an extra squirt of grease to keep the joints from rusting, but that's small beans for the view I'll get from the tops of the mountains I've yet to climb and the food I have yet to taste in countries and worlds I have yet to traverse. Heck, I still have to figure out what you women folk are all about, although generations past have confided in me that you will probably always remain the greatest of scary and wonderful mysteries. I like mysteries.

Does any of this seem easier to accomplish if my machine isn't kept purring?

A quick glance around my neighborhood seems to confirm the guess that some of my peers have already stored their carriages in the garage, covering them until the day seems right to dust it off, if that day ever comes. A daily scene directly outside my shanty features my neighbor rapidly inhaling his 20th or so cigarette of that day. He is so slouched over that his frail, emaciated frame looks like he's permanently stooping below doorframes, which he'd better hold onto so the breeze doesn't blow him away.

He's 22. Not only is there not enough of a past to truly demand this posture and ill health of his, there will be no future except that which will enhance it. He's not alone either. His clan is everywhere, a tribe without longevity, Darwinism on display if you're willing enough to watch it. Silly me... you're eager to get moving, aren't you?

I'm personally faced with a dichotomy. Look, as I mosh my way through my 5th decade, I haven't yet donned the garments that seem trendy with my chronological peers. Not married, no children, and a career that can be fodder for an SNL skit (or an entire movie... remember Dodgeball?). I've been ducking responsibility like a ninja since I first rolled off the diaper-changing table and ran out in the yard nekkid and laughing (sure, that might have been last Thursday, but you get the idea).

Watching a generation replace choices of responsibility (or the lack of, in my case) with the bondage of addictions and dilapidated health is like flipping through a chose-your-own-ending book that only has one chapter.

Movement, health, and longevity all share similar DNA. Where does an individual lose touch with movement?

I remember the day I cried because my overweight friend Lynn broke my big wheel. At the time I missed the relevance of the event... kudos to Lynn for riding the crap out of that thing until it could no longer bear her larger than average size. Sure enough, Lynn went on to ride bigger rigs that could sustain her mass, and the Gods of correlation giggled because the more she rode, played, and behaved with the intent of having fun, the more her mass shrunk. She pulled out of her foray into double digit chronology with a much more reasonable weight-to-height ratio before I lost track of her.

Then there's "Jay". In early High School, Jay was my dichotomous close friend - he liked Christian rock while I listened to Slayer; he lifted weights and had a collection of team letters while I ran from the jocks so they didn't beat me up; he was college bound and career ready while I was wondering which fast food hat looked best with my long hair.

Thanks to Facebook, I now know Jay's stats are... well, let's just say considerably different. Obviously overweight and out of shape, his choices make me again wonder...

Where did he lose touch with movement?

Our American school system seems to work like this...

1-12 years old: go ahead and play. We'll give you a sliver of time called recess, and then if you were lucky, you had a bit of freedom after school. Don't worry, rules aren't important yet, but you'd better start learning them soon (heck, look 'em up on your phone), because...

13-18 years of age: you've got two choices... pick a sport or stop playing entirely. Unfortunately, sport is not synonymous with play, no matter what the AYSO propaganda states. Now is the time to covet winning, not playing. If you're good enough, you might get to do more of it in college. Otherwise, this might be your last dance with organized movement for many years.

19-22 years of age. Do you play a sport?

Yes = possible over-training and burnout from competition, with a HUGE chance that after college you may never want to 'play' again.

No = you won't start now. If you're lucky, you might start working out a little, especially if you believe, like many do, that it will help you get laid. Welcome to obligatory movement. No play to be found here.

23- onward... "Working out" replaces actual movement and play. Now movement is exercise, an obligation through redundant reps and limited ranges of movement. What was once a tension release as a child is now building more tension to your already full arsenal.

Almost daily I meet folks (like myself) who have been through some version of this timeline. Either movement is loaded onto our shoulders like a yoke of obligation as we age, or we avoid it entirely. Sound off with me, folks... how do we make changes to that?

Make some noise! Welcome back to playtime! Be ridiculous, be intense, a little brutal, and a bunch of wonderful. THAT'S what movement is meant to be, and we should NEVER lose sight of that!

In the words of Tom Waits, I don't wanna grow up. At least my body doesn't. Better decisions now for more choices later. Simply put, better the Now to enhance the Later.

16. Are You Happy?

Remember the second part of our Transformation recipe? Consistency! First the joy of intensity, then repeat it.

We're born with potential. Our latent abilities are what separates us from the other fauna on the planet, and that ain't meant as a boost to the esteem of our species. Other animals meet their potential pretty quickly through preset software. We're factory installed with only a blank map, an empty guidebook, and a big metaphysical machete, and if your tribe does its job of lurnin' you right, then you'll end up pretty darn skilled at using that machete to chop through the jungle of nonsense.

We're manufactured from some DNA that demands a daily gallon or so of blood, sweat, toil, tears, passion, curiosity (possibly outright fear), and tenacity to glean to most out of our flesh packets. We're machines of a special type. Organic, biological. Not quite the perfect movers that some of the recent training protocols are hoping we are. In other words, we are not built for many of the workouts advocated (read: sold) for bodies, at least not without some serious practice and training. The high rep workload trend seems to forget that crucial little point that I mentioned Tommy Kono regularly drilled into our heads every time he visited BodyTribe:

Practice makes PERMANENT.

If your gym life is the extent of your movement life, you've become a full-blown adult. There is no congratulations attached to this fact, since, frankly, you're biding your time. The one purpose of your body, how your hylomorphic package finds joy and success, is movement, and you've relegated it to a job, a chore. All fun stripped out of it as it becomes a tick on your checklist.

Let's remember joy. All the other movement choices we can make, from dance to sport to recreational adventure, to stuff reserved for behind closed doors, is all about the quest for joy. Deeply satisfying movement. Not only do we often forget about these never ending options, but we reduce our movement choices to the walls of a gym, to the categories of the fitness industry, to the adult-brained version of fitness.

Movement should be a gateway drug, an exponential philosophy where one choice begets many more. Darn our adult brains and the control they want to have over our bodies.

Let's chat a bit about how we sabotage our movement potential through physical and philosophical mythologies the brain has created about movement and exercise, and how to free ourselves from them.

Chasing Exhaustion

I don't care how you workout near as much as how you live! If you live to workout, perhaps you've got it backwards. I dig your 800 pound squat, but I really want to see what that is doing for you.

Now every time I mention the concept of training as a means to get better at physical skills, folks all emphatically nod in agreement... but then run off to conquer their 50 burpee-ups and 100 bend-and-snaps and 200 kegal-outs. This trend seems to indicate the only skill anyone wants to improve is their ability to work out harder.

In a great majority of workshops I teach, I'm in front of groups of people where possibly everyone in the room could out-workout me. On every given day they could WOD all over me. Maybe they'd bootcamp me right into the ground. In the our workshop, though, I'll spend the next 2-5 hours showing them what they can't do, or at least what they could do better, simply by implementing strict foundations of proper movement into their exercise choices. Most importantly, they'll learn how to take that gym stuff and go get a life with it. I don't care that you can cram in a bunch of reps in a shorter time period than I can. I'd like to show you that skill is built differently. It's not acquired just by chasing exhaustion.

Because 'fitness' has a byproduct of being tired, we've turned it into the goal. Now there are two camps of chasing exhaustion:

1. Chase the fatigue to conquer the fatigue.

The skill of not pooping out as easily. In other words, push the constitutional boundaries into the red so there is a greater foundation for work capacity when practicing other skills. We could find some serious validity to this, and in the ol' days, before it got the fancy name of 'metabolic conditioning,' we called it GPP, general physical preparedness. It was used not only to have a grounding in increased stamina for further skill building, but a blanket ability of being a good beginner at any skill. In other words, it's going through kindergarten in skill potential.

I've already mentioned where it has gone awry. The trending belief now is that this is THE skill to have, so the majority of intensity in the gym is geared to doing MORE FASTER, forever building the skill of working out by conditioning the ability to fight the fatigue of that workout. Does it seem wise to use important movement skills of some degree of difficulty for that conditioning, even if it means actually letting those skills break down?

Here is a very common story, although names are changed to protect the victims of modern fitness propaganda:

An extreme exhaustion chaser, we'll call him David Lee

Roth[9], and I were chatting recently. A sweet guy and a frenetic energy ball, he was regaling me with tales of yesterday's extreme WOD, followed by that morning's other extreme WOD. All the ass got kicked and all the sweat puddled and spilled. This day was far from the first time I had heard these exclamations of his quest for lung-shattering, muscle burning workouts. In fact, it is sort of his thing. Facebook and social media are his popular outlets for AMRAPs and buy-ins and EMOMs (yep, if you're new to this, bust out your Trendy-Workout-to-English dictionary now. Actually, nah, don't bother.), and the hundreds of reps and rounds he routinely attacks. Chasing exhaustion is a big part of his identity.

It takes me less than a minute to show him something he can't do.

I don't produce the greatest mega-workout for him to try, nor am I any kind of super athlete with mad skills to show off. I just offer some playtime, and playtime actually requires some basic movement skills that aren't taught much, or don't even seem to be coveted, in our live-to-workout industry. Nothing in his WODtastic, 'functional' training actually gave him the skills to just move and play. He can sweat circles around me (he actually competes in this stuff), but he hasn't built too many usable skills or abilities that I have found to lead to even greater skill chunks. What's his end game?

A 'functional' exercise can be completely voided by sloppy programming.

Within our transformation recipe, Consistency sans Purpose is incomplete.

2. Chasing exhaustion as an addiction.

Recently I heard Doug Kraft speak and lead a meditation here in Sacramento. Part of his talk expanded on something I've

---

[9] No, not his real name. But in surprising rockstar trivia twist: it is David Lee Roth's real name.

heard before. When spiritual leaders visit from other countries, they are often surprised and shocked by how much we seem to hate ourselves, and how it shows itself in various forms of abuse. Strange how I had examples right on the edge of my noggin of people I've experienced over the years who have treated their movement journeys as struggle fests. Many folks with this specific personality trait have bought into this modern beat-your-ass-up workout world because, simply, they're addicted to abuse. Whether chemical, emotional, or the very tactile, physical abuse of poor training programming, we have a growing culture of perpetuation of this tweaked idea of body relations, and the modern gym culture is not helping. In fact we celebrate it. From screwed up ideals like websites called Live Sore[10] to the popular pump up vernacular strewn with clichés like Extreme or Beast Mode, the take away seems to be that we're not doing it right unless we create some unbalanced relationship with our bodies where the brain is the master, and the body is the slave. Ironically, that's actually the opposite of how addiction really works ... but you can see the dichotomy that an addict will find appealing in our world of trumpeted self-abuse.

Your gym most likely has at least one of these people, but cognitive dissonance, supported by a culture that clicks that 'like' button every time he or she posts a picture of themselves in a sweat puddle on the floor, assures them that it is a coveted ideal.

Obsession is dysfunction, parading falsely as passion.

Meanwhile the dual edge of the battle axe that is the internet helps build a bigger community while also perpetuating the flaws that ultimately can destroy our world wide tribe. In the case of our current topic, social media allows us to mistake chasing exhaustion for skill building. We smear

---

[10] A friend wondered why a website would celebrate an open wound. He thought it was pronounced "live' as in 'a live studio audience.'

our facetubestagram with videos of highly skilled movement and strength artists, lauding them as shining examples of human achievement. Yes. Yes they are. They might even be a delicious part of our inspiration breakfast.

Then off to the gym we go, beating ourselves up by doing redundant reps of our same basic-level skills over and over, somehow believing it's sort of the same thing. Splashing paint all over a canvas until you're thoroughly spent is not the same league as creating a masterpiece

'Functional' training ruined by dysfunctional programming. Now trending.

17. Repeating Preschool Won't Get You into High School
(Intensity through Planning)

A toddler picks up a stick and whacks it against a box. Thwack. He giggles. *Thwack*Thwack*Thwack* A new skill is born, and he's excited.

Hey mom! *Thwack*

Mooooom!!! *Thwack*Thwack*Thwack*

Mom, look! Mom! Mom, look at meeee!

*Thwack*Thwack*Thwack*Thwack *Thwack*Thwack*

Fast-forward 20 years. An adult learns the muscle-up[11]...

Up... hey look....*Up*Up*Up*

Hey mom! *Up*Up*Up*

Hey internet... look at meeee! *Up*Up*Up*Up*

The difference is that toddler will quickly move on to a new skill. Once he groks that he can beat the crap out of that box just fine, it's time to explore more of life. He can now run the stick across fences, throw it over things, maybe even swing it around like a certain barbarian warrior. Thwacking stuff isn't increasing his skill base anymore, and it's a big world out there.

---

[11] Remember these from the Potential versus Actual Strength chapter?

The adult, on the other hand, decides if one muscle up is good, 10 are better. And they should be done faster. And maybe they should even be competitive. Oh, and 20 are even better than that. Thwack*thwack.

Here's why the adult lost his way. As we mentioned chapters ago, the muscle up is kindergarten ring work, and it has one purpose... to get up on the rings to do other things. Maybe continually practicing to get up on the rings is time better spent actually pursuing the next round of skills. The kid with a stick eventually explored where he could go with that stick, and life became way more interesting. Something in our adult brain, on the other hand, turns movement into a task, not a celebration of possibility.

You can do a few in a row? Time to graduate. Now you're up there... what can you do? Adding more and more to that set of muscle ups is not building any more skill; it's chasing exhaustion. Doing more for the only outcome of getting tired doing that one thing. We can spice up the sales pitch with all the catchy, important-sounding words we want, like 'power output' or 'work capacity.' The reality is less exciting. You're just repeating a lower level skill to beat yourself up. That's time wasted.

If we're aiming for increased skill (which I thought we all agreed upon as our goal), then the hierarchy of climbing up on stuff might go something like this. Can you hang from a bar? Groovy. You're a climbing toddler. Can you do some pull-ups? Superb, you're in climbing preschool. That muscle up puts you in climbing kindergarten, where you can begin planning for a bevy of things that you can eventually do once you're ready to work yourself up to the higher grade levels of getting up, on, and then over, stuff.

The current model enjoys being stuck mastering preschool or kindergarten. Sort of seems a bit redundant, doesn't it? 1 pull-up is a good start, 10 unbroken pull-ups seems like a good progression, but 30 pull-ups in a row? Sure... as the outcome of already being a great climber or gymnast, perhaps, but as the *outcome*... not the goal. Once you work your way up the skill chart, then being able to do 30 pull-ups would be *a result* of building other more important skills. Having 30 pull-ups AS a goal DOES NOT graduate you any higher up that skill chart. Why repeat preschool? Mastering basic math over and over again doesn't give you mad algebra skills.

How do we change our current paradigm? Let's talk more about skill building as job 1.

18. Skills

I ain't too bright. It's been said that if something can't be explained to a child, then its worth, heck, its existence, is questionable. I say Amen. Consider me that child.

I say movement isn't that complicated. In fact, here are some groovy concepts to chew on...

1) Your body learns movement faster then your brain.

2) Your body wants to move. In more ways than your brain can imagine.

3) The body listens to the brain, even when the information is contrary to the body's purpose. Sometimes the brain has to shut its damn mouth.

Too bad our brains work in many ways to jeopardize the body and what it is made for. One of those ways is to market movement and strength. Our brains seem to believe that to sell movement, we have to limit it and package it. Now this, in itself, isn't always a bad thing. Our brains, however, will then crave a little validation. Suddenly we need to tell other brains that there should be no other options. Buy our package! The others don't count. Once again the message screams *our way of exercising is better than what you're doing*! Buy it.

Or maybe the brain chooses a tool or program and simply ignores other options. Hey, we all have preferences for genres, and certain styles and gadgets can often dominate our attention. We can all be seduced by something amazing. Just keep an eye out for that *dogma biting your ass-ma*. Dig what you wanna dig, but let your stubbornness relax so some other forms of awesomeness might permeate its shield. A great deal of what you aren't embracing might even support what you love (and a great deal of what you're currently doing might be keeping you distracted).

The Authentic Athlete understands that movement is what the body, this glorious organic machine we're all given, is for, and that the point of that movement is to form a relationship with mind, soul, planet, and tribe. Join me, will you, in exploring what our machines do. Let's start at the beginning...

Your Human Experience, Day One and Beyond:

Congrats! You're born. Can't do much yet though. Heck, you don't even have fully formed kneecaps. But as a little bundle of humanness you still crave discovering your place on this planet. Walking and talking are so far away as to be unreal, but you will still participate, damn it! Your arms and legs and fingers and toes and feet and hands will go anywhere they can... in there, over there, around there, up there.

We begin our quest to experience life with movement. Our skills, though, are admittedly, pretty basic. We're not deterred! We take what little freedom we have and we're going with it. Experimenting with space and filling up as much of it as we can with the little we've got. We're *flowing*, baby, and this movement stuff is not only important, it's glorious! We're using the little we have to the utmost potential, and because of our desire to take up space, to extend our range, we progress. We grow.

The big bummer is that as we gain the potential for so many more movement discovery options later in life, we actually limit ourselves into adulthood. Not the body's choice, these limitations, by the way. Let's remember that.

Half way through the first year:

   Knees in, curiosity on, and muscles forming, this spinning space machine called earth has more to offer us. We add direction to the fairly stationary flow we've had up until this point. Hands and feet are now our own personal wheels, and kiddo, we're going for a ride. What's over there? Under here? Around that? Who are you? Can I move this? We can start answering these questions. Movement is knowledge, damn it! We're crawling, learning mechanisms and, again, the constant striving to increase our potential allows us to grow, literally and then some.

   What's up there? *Crawl*, grab, pull, struggle... and *Fall*. This exploration, and occasional failure, allows the muscles to strengthen, and our bodies begin to understand directional relationships even more. Movement is wisdom... and Strength!

75% through the first year:

   Falling was fun and all, but not falling by having a bit more reliance on these two chubby planks under our butt seems important. If we bend them, we can hang out in this upright, seated position for a while. In a few decades we'll look back with envy at these mad squat skills, but for now we're still trying to simply not fall over. We're now beginning to dream of going somewhere on just 2 wheels instead of 4. We need to continue to practice our ability to *Rise*.

   The first year ends with us in the upright boogie. *Standing*! Holy cow, have you seen what we accomplished in the first year? We're up, and moving! Suck it, gravity. Who's the boss now?

   It has been said that we learn more in the first 2-3 years of life than we will the rest of our lives combined. Movement, and acquiring the strength to move, is not just a big part of that process... it IS that process. Movement is the tactile experience of the planet. Let's not let that go to waste as our chronology (and sometimes waistband) expands. Move and learn.

Skills. That's what our movement practice is all about. Being able to do stuff towards our greater purpose of being useful. Understanding how the modern fitness paradigm relishes redundancy and exhaustion isn't tough. The status quo of entertaining the masses into being tired, usually for aesthetic gain, is antithetical to striving to be able to DO anything. Somehow our mastery of cognitive dissonance keeps the belief alive that exercise and skill building are synonymous.

They should be. Through the common workout beliefs and tenets currently being bought and sold, they're not.

Let's make the physical purpose for training to be skill building. We can use the example of our first year of life above to create a solid list of the Big Picture Skill Chunks. These are the umbrellas that everything we learn can fall under. We should be finding a balance in our skills, filling these categories evenly and, ultimately, with purpose. Our path to usefulness will have us continually working towards being able to...

Stand
Rise
Fall
Crawl
and **Flow**.

Stand: Simple (because that's how I like it). Skills on two legs (or two arms, if we go upside down... yes, for reals). This skill chunk takes care of movements of running, walking, carrying, picking stuff up...Anything where the body is upright, creating support, flux, and stabilization from a standing, upright position (even if it is upside down).

Rise: The process of going higher. Changing elevation, which might be getting up from the floor, or the hinging and straightening of the knees and hips (if you guessed squatting, lunging, deadlift, etc... you win!), and also includes climbing... getting up and down off of something.

Fall: Oh, a brilliant category that is so often ignored. The skill of absorbing force. Landing, catching and, of course, actually falling. This might be the most forgotten category for adults. I recently had someone tell me that this category was superfluous because it was a muscle action, sometimes known as explosive or accelerated eccentric action, therefor not a skill. Not a skill? Two important things to consider... we all need to understand how to do it, and most folks can't. Ask any martial arts instructor... I'll bet they've got stories of how any beginner doesn't know how to land or fall. At BodyTribe we work on the basics of falling almost immediately as a foundation to so much of movement... but we'll get to that in a bit.

Crawl: Be on the ground and do stuff there. These days this category gets press with the recent focus on 'primal' movements. Labeling movement 'primal' just seems like a fancy way of selling 'human,' but with connection to a different chronology. That just gets too confusing. You wouldn't tell a child that crawling, rolling and tumbling are primal. To them, that's just what the body does, among other things. Crawling, as a skill category, is getting connected to the ground using as many body parts as you can. If all the limbs are involved in connecting to the ground, it falls in this category. From very real crawling, to pushups, tumbling, and a handful of asanas.

Flow: Flow is three important things:

> 1) The ability to transition, or 'morph' as we'll call it, between shapes.

> 2) Moving with grace and mastery. Your strength is not complete if it doesn't lead to good movement patterns.

No matter how great your range of motion becomes, your mobility is lacking if the quality and beauty in the movements resemble an evil robot from a 50s sci-fi movie. If you hanker for a James Cameron reference, (and who doesn't?), think T-1000 rather than the 800 series... but without the constant mission to purge the earth of human life.

3) Exploration. This is where we grow, as humans, through the experimentation of where we are in space... just like the infant example not too long ago. Without exploration our bodies will miss their potential, no matter how good we are in the gym.

Many folks I've had the honor of working with find that breathing seems to be an important skill on its own. Absolutely. I'd put it under this Flow header.

Flow is where we start as humans, yet it is the skill we will spend the rest of our lives attempting to master. Visually it could be the circle that all the other Big Picture Skill Chunks are wrapped up in.

Oh yes, I'm sure your adult brain is creating all sorts of additional categories (chunks) already ("what about throw?" "There's always jumping"). I'll bet they'll fit nicely as a subcategory of any of these 5 Big Picture Skill Chunks. If that just chaps your hide, if you crave stats and heavy analysis and the days when you memorized everything Gary Gygax[12] ever wrote, then by all means, create your massive, cross-referenced and complicated skill list. But this is simple human movement. As we've explored, this list is how we learn movement from day one, although backwards from how I list it here.

---

[12] Serious nerd points if that reference had you ready to roll to save against polymorph.

But where do we begin?

We now have an idea of where we're headed, practicing skills within a balanced program that will flesh out the Big Picture Skill Chunks. But first we've got something important to deal with, something that is horribly mishandled by the current Fitness Industrial Complex. What are the actual foundations? Where do we start?

Watering down athletic programs for the masses seems to be the rage right now. Train like a hardcore athlete... but not quite. CrossFit, MMA training, and endless other programs offered through the nouveau fitness culture highlight how effective they are for serious athletes... but don't worry, we've got a version for you too. We'll water it down for you average folks, and smooth them out even more for those beginners out there.

This is completely backwards. What we're discovering at BodyTribe is how we *all* need a place to begin, no matter how long you've been involved in this training stuff. Which, therefore, might mean starting a new journey.

Becoming a specialized athlete can easily mean skipping important steps of understanding actual movement. We're masters at compensation. Our bodies will make up for these missed steps by gaining the ability through faulty movement patterns. Then, to 'master' our sport of choice, we'll excel at these faulty movement patterns.

In other words, even great athletes need to learn how to move. Instead of promoting athletic training programs as the path for everyone, even with the diluted options, let's create an entirely new paradigm.

First, and here's a biggie, let's learn movement before we practice exercise. We should also work on understanding the difference.

These days this 'movement' concept has become its own packaged category. Call it the primal natural animal trend. We sure do have a soft spot for romanticizing simplicity. Or maybe we're just trying to make a buck.

Anyway, to understand our own movement philosophy, we're faced with a surprisingly tough challenge:

How simple can we make it?

I'm going to posit that our quest for ability (you know... strength) also means improving our skills from a basic foundation of how to...

Roll
Crawl
Change Elevation (get up and down)
Pick Stuff Up
Put Stuff Overhead
Carry stuff

Always answering the question: if there is an obstacle in our way, can we get over it, around it, under it, through it or move it? Let's start thinking "yes" to all of them. Doesn't get more 'primal/natural/animal' (simple) than that.

Or it might. Our entire practice is simplified even further...

Get Up
Get Down
Move It
Groove it

This dancehall cliché might be my motto for any movement practice. We're can spend the rest of our lives perpetually exploring from this premise. Get up (and do stuff up there), get down (and do stuff down there), move it (yourself or something else), groove it (do it all well).

So, to have an infrastructure from which to build on, back to this list...

Roll
Crawl
Change Elevation
Pick Stuff Up
Put Stuff Overhead
Carry stuff

In reading that list, you might observe a few things. First, it doesn't look particularly dissimilar to the Big Picture Skill Chunk list. Don't worry, that's a good thing.

Second, if we've had any gym experience, we've probably put movement ideas to some of these. Pick up stuff? Heck, that's a deadlift. Putting stuff over our heads? That's a press. Hold on... we'll get there.

As you expand your mastering of the foundations, you can graduate to building a repertoire in the Big Picture Skill Chunks. The problem is, in our quest for cool, in our dreams of fame, or simply because we want some throbbing biceps and a million hits on our Instagram pic, we often skip the foundations and work on specializing. We all know a handful of skilled athletes or veteran gym rats who are less than capable in some of these basics.

You and your creative head and passionate soul can begin defining what these mean by assigning movements to them. Shucks, you might even come up with your own foundation list. Without a place to start, though, without a baseline standard, whether it's this one, or one of your own, you'll struggle for completeness. Which, frankly, might not be the goal of a great many people steeped in a superficial idea of exercise. Remember... our purpose here is usefulness

The gist of the BodyTribe template is to teach and perpetuate these foundations, which always feed the Big Picture Skill Chunks.

Setting the lowest bar, and then raising it

In programming, gym veterans often set benchmarks... be able to squat double bodyweight or toss a baby 100 feet or punch through a narwhal hide with your pinkie. We like benchmarks. Our brains crave standards, so we look for ideas of where our potential should be. Dan John says if a woman can deadlift 275 pounds, the performance world opens up to her, for instance.

To simplify all this, decide what you believe foundation skills are, or borrow mine above. Yup. For free. No certification required.

If you're a trainer, ask yourself what everyone in your tribe should be able to do and continuing to improve upon. Then decide what the lowest foundation is that you'll accept. In other words, what should everyone in your tribe, *no matter what*, be able to do? This substratum of skills isn't an entrance exam, though. They simply indicate the movement bedrock of your programming. If someone lacks any of these skills, you, as their movement sherpa, have some work to do.

Then you can build levels. If they can do the foundation skills at level A, how about B? You might discover that some folks who can level F a certain skill all day, will be barely proficient at a level B of another skill. Guess where their weak points are? Which is why, surprisingly, you might find the beginners aren't always the ones you have to keep an eye on. Specialized athletes often skip this basic foundation concept for something shinier, like a bigger clean and jerk or higher Girevoy Sport[13] numbers, while bypassing some basic skills in the process. This performance focus often leads to unbalanced potential.

Now we've mentioned the Foundation Skills. Here a rundown of what they mean, and where level A begins:

---

[13] An endurance event based around kettlebells and questionable posture.

Roll: Basic knowledge of engaging the ground. Being so low to terra firma is surprisingly hard for even advanced athletes who haven't played this way in a while. Level A: just a simple backwards and forwards cradle rock, holding onto the knees.

Crawl: Being able to move on all fours. Level A: an actual crawl on the hands and knees.

Change Elevation: Getting up, and also getting back down. The level A standard here is to be able to get up and down off the floor, get in and out of a chair, get up and down from a 36″ plinth or box (not jumping, just getting on and off it), and a good 30 second hang from a bar. Yeah, there are many ways to get up on things. We, animals of exploration, may want to consider them all.

Pick something up: This skill is the ability to pick something up (what did you expect?). Level A: be able to pick something up. Yes, it's that simple. In this case, weight doesn't enter the equation with any importance. Simply knowing the proper mechanics is the goal. If you ever watch powerlifting competitions, you may notice many have skipped level A, letting the weight on the bar trump useable skill. Oops.

Put something overhead: Now the first thought you may have is 'overhead press.' Sure, but for a big chunk of our society (both fit and unfit) they lack the correct shoulder and back prowess (be it weakness or tightness) to pull this off safely. Consider other options like club work, or even simple arm circles, for a more appropriate for level A.

Carry something: Seems pretty basic, right? It is. For you trainer geeks who bore your clients to tears with technical jargon, call this loaded terra-based upright biomobile kinetics(tm). Heck, just be well versed in all the potential ways to actually carry stuff. The foundation of this skill is to have at least one option under the belt. By the way, sometimes all we need to carry is ourselves. Just being upright and getting from point A to Point B could constitute carrying something.

Always continuing to grow in proficiency in the foundations will add to our Big Picture Skill Chunks, and skipping any of these will be a noticeable gap in overall ability.

Now you've probably already begun assigning movements to this list. Pick something up? That's a deadlift, you say! You wouldn't be wrong. Now your next goal is to choose the movements you feel best represent each foundation. So many choices! Get moving. Are you a collection of exercises, or are your movements improving your Big Picture Skill Chunks?

19. Do Better
(Intensity through Purity)

Move *well,* and you'll learn well. Move poorly, and you'll learn poorly. Move productively... well, you get the idea. Your lessons will reflect your movement choices. If we're busy just to be busy, as is quite common in the fitness world right now, then the lessons are minimal.

Movement with purpose, *strength with intent...*your humanness becomes defined. You Become, not just exist.

Do it right. Before you do it more, do it better. Priority number 1. Oh, many a workshop I have taught where simply correcting pushup form reduced everyone's numbers into low double digits, or even single digits. Oh... and it makes the workout even harder.

Look... a hard, crappy workout is still a crappy workout. Enduring a tough workout is not life changing. Enduring a *good* workout is, but it can be a struggle finding a modern fit pro who knows the difference. The false empowerment of accomplishing a poorly executed workout is currently fueling the nouveau fitness culture, creating the belief that surviving some sort of grueling mishmash of challenging exercises, through any means necessary, is the only goal worth having.

If practice makes permanent, and by now you know it does, then the current beat-the-stopwatch model of 'do a lot, fast' is teaching our organic machines slop, therefore making slop permanent. And that breaks machines. Workload is an important factor in fitness, but it is not the ONLY factor by far, nor does it have to be sloppy. Volume and speed are only two ingredients to an athletic stew, and any true coach worth a damn understands that these ingredients are malleable. More of either or both is not always the best option. Often, BETTER is the most important element to making us better. More technique, not volume or speed, can add an intensity challenge and embodiment quality that has a greater effect on the human body. Repeat that into mastery (remember the second part of **Transformation** is Consistency).

Your body needs you to believe that doing something correctly is Job One. Let's talk about why.

I've been as guilty as the next gym for being cutesy with creating themed workouts, but I can't keep up with the true artists of mayhem. My social media feed is littered with concepts like a 50 Shades of WOD workout that had 50 reps of 12 different exercises. These chosen exercises are usually the common popular culprits of wall balls, pushups, air squats, etc... the standard nouveau–fitness arsenal that has infiltrated so many programs.

I might be preaching heretical thinking, but I rarely need to know that my athletes can do 50 of almost anything in a row. In all the workshops I've taught, even to big rooms of trainers, I've seen what 10 pushups looks like to the vast majority of people. I can only imagine what 50 will do. Add burpees to that mix... have emergency crews standing by!

That 50 rep set of pushups might see a handful of something that might be called a pushup towards the beginning... maybe, just maybe 10 do actually look good. Then the next 40 might turn into slop, just because you're under the clock and gotta do those 50 with the goal of speed trumping all else. This isn't program design. 10 pushups that might help the body, and 40 that suck... a 400% practice of slop.

Once again, practice makes permanent... guess what you're practicing? Add a barbell to this type of party and things have an even greater chance of going wonky. If the goal is to build skill, which I thought we agreed on, then it seems that yanking the bar from the ground to your chest 30+ times in a row must make you better at something. But what? High rep bar yanking while competing against a stopwatch will have no real chance of making you a more skilled Olympic lifter. We shouldn't even compare it to Olympic lifting technique. It's a new beast, and the impact on your organic machine might demand questioning as to why you're doing it.

For a book that stated it wasn't going to mention program design much, this book sure mentions program design a lot. Oops. How about a challenge? If intensity through purity (meaning doing a movement better) is our first goal, then what might be second? Volume and speed are still not considerations yet, at least as a pairing. We can do more... just as long as the equation is do more, better. We can be faster... as long as the movement is precise and well executed. We have better options than putting the two together.

We've listed some of the other possibilities already. A good coach has a list of malleable factors they can manipulate to up the intensity. Quality of movement should top the list. Load, positioning, distance, speed, duration, tool choice, and volume are all on that list. If we're limited to the marriage of speed and volume, we're limited as a trainer or movement educator.

Without turning this into a holistic program design manual, here's your homework assignment: You have 10 pushups. How could you make these 10 pushups more beneficial than 50? You don't get to increase the number.

Let's begin the thought process with this: for most people, 50 would get sloppy, fast. Heck, from my experience, even with advanced fitness folks, 10 or 15 often gets sloppy fast.

More is just a number, a quantity. Better is actually a quality. Let's focus on quality first. How can we make these pushups better? Better for you and your organic machine. Better for further skill development. Better for your hylomorphic self. A considerably bigger process than adding more reps faster.

20. Dancing Monkey Syndrome
(Intensity Through Philosophy)

I'm often reminded that information exchange in this industry of exercise is often less cognitive and far more corporeal. Which, initially, makes sense, but then there lies the major fallacy of this industrial complex.

This industry teaches exercise, but has a hard time exploring movement.

Try to add the philosophy of purpose to that, and ears cover with callused hands quickly to the tune of lalalalala, I can't hear you. This education gap seems to be why a 8 second clip of a deadlift gets more attention than, say, 160-page book about the purpose of training.

I have detractors. Weird, right? One of them pops up somewhere in the comments section of my various social media expressions, especially if anything in the discussion seems to, even vaguely, point a finger, or even a toe, at his favorite training protocol as something that could be done better. Instead of the philosophical banter one can hope for, if there was some, a common formula unfolds. The I-post/he-reacts/I-elaborate/ he-disappears model.

Can you guess what elicits a positive response from this brand of critic? There is a category of expression common in the virtual world that I call the Dancing Monkey video. It's a short clip, usually no words, of some movement or strength feat. I rarely post them. A lesson, or at least a good rant, seems more conducive to my soul, so I often elaborate on an idea until it becomes a 2-hour DVD or 4-part downloadable series. I'm compelled to add some substance, which is why there are very few videos under 10 minutes long on the BodyTribe YouTube channel[14]. To see a quick, basic, today-I-did-this video of mine enter the internet-o-sphere is a rare thing. Fear not. Everyone else seems to be making a lot of them, and probably better than I can. You'll still get your fix.

There is another reason they don't often flow from my practice into the public. Immediately after I post a snippet video of the aforementioned ilk, the response from those said detractors is often "YES! That's what I love about what you do. Show us more of that!" Strangely, I feel a little icky afterwards.

In this nouveau fitness culture of play and flow, often with the hyperbolic label "primal," being labeled a dancing monkey would seem complimentary. Even ideal. But the term is pejorative, portraying the concept of obedient servant. That comment on my post may as well have read 'dance, monkey, dance.'

I ramble. My pie hole may not be impressive in size or power (like most of me). But in volume, this mouth of mine has tenacity to its ability to wax diatribally (which my spell check says isn't a word, but it also has a problem with 'deadlift,' so what does it know?).

The brain and body jig with the heart in a perpetual meringue of contemplating a little meaning to it all. Perhaps my output comes across as crass, especially when a distracting trend or cliché begins washing a bunch of brains and I happen

---

[14] www.youtube.com/user/Bodytribe1, by the way.

to call it out. Dogmas get frazzled.

Once in awhile, there is the honor of being a conduit for potential. When a door is kicked down by my size 42 Feiyues, every now and then I'm joined by a few other pairs of eyes (and shoes) to explore what's beyond it. My insides find a spiritual joy when I see my own words in a post or a meme (often anonymously quoted, but so what?) put out into the universe (well... interwebular galaxy) by someone I might barely know beyond a 'like' or two on Facebook.

Sometimes my words find spiritual kin, which can cultivate into something a little magical. Maybe a workshop tour comes together for some folks who have taken to kicking down similar doors, or at least being there when my heel did the work. My path then connects with a host of other seekers, teaching, and of course learning, all headed to the top of the same proverbial mountain.

I write and rant and enter a handful of dialogs about movement or exercise as a needed outlet for the non-corporeal part of my hylomorphic self. In other words, I feel we gotta talk this out, because, as we've been discussing throughout this book, there are a big bunch of folks who are lacking purpose in their exercise, and an even bigger bunch who aren't moving at all. I crave purpose, always attempting to answer that perpetual question: Am I useful?

Perhaps you can hear the giant sucking sound where this sort of banter ought to exist. We might hear a little chatter, a barely detectable dialog, like a hum that makes our tiny ear hairs lightly bristle. But hardly any of the modern fitness dialog moves beyond the Me, Me, look at Me selfie culture. We're so busy talking about how great we are at working out, we forgot how meaningless that workout probably is in big-picture, wide-angle lens format. You've got this amazing program that you bought into... so what?

Point being, I find the philosophy of movement often more important than the demonstration of it, simply because everyone is already talking about the What and the How. What to do and How to do it fills every nook and cranny of the fitness world's social media. If you question the *Why*, though, sometimes hell breaks loose. Purpose simply isn't the thing people want to talk about.

No matter how badly we need to be asking Why, we still suffer from Dancing Monkey Syndrome. Most people will tolerate my ranting with polite nods, or they'll get frisky in their disagreement until they run out of steam, but post a video of a groovy little movement creation and the Dancing Monkey Syndrome kicks in. I've been brought to gyms in the past so they could simply take whatever cool new moves I happened to show them, while they gently endured my philosophical blabbering. I was their dancing monkey. I get it... that's what we do. Teach exercise. Look at the dancing monkey... then replicate it.

There is our failure, or at least my lack of understanding. I'm not a particularly skilled athlete, but in most workshops I impart a great deal of new movement ideas to the participants. I'm grateful for this privilege, but I have a caveat. Next time I come through, show me what you've done with this information. The movement ideas are simply an expression of my philosophy of exploration and play, how strength in action should look. When I'm surrounded by a room full of people who can out-workout me, my hope is that I'm offering the artist's rendering of what the purpose of working out is... the foundation of building skills. This monkey will dance, demonstrating what these skills in action might look like, then I'll talk in length about why a workout is meaningless unless there is a point to it. I'll look on the surrounding white boards and see all the times and weights posted by members of that gym, and usually rank myself in the bottom half of what I see. Then I'll show you where your strength might go, what it might look like in action, and being allowed access to freedom of movement is always a little surprising to everyone.

I'm not a dancing monkey showing you the newest trick. I'm showing you a philosophy of strength as action. Steal the moves if you'd like... they weren't mine to begin with. What is your journey? I've walked many paths, always to bring back the fruits of my own freshly trod quest. You can simply mimic me, or any of the videos from whatever movement mentor you've chosen to emulate. Then who is the dancing monkey?

21. The Tribe Section
(Intensity through Community)

Would you just take, along with me, 10 seconds to think of the people who helped you become who you are. Those who have cared about you and wanted what was best for you in life. 10 seconds. I'll watch the time.
— Fred Rogers.

What is Tribe?

When you're 11, about as socially adequate as a stripper at a bar mitzvah, and blessed with skills and intelligence that could be certified as 'strongly average,' the quest for a peer group might lead you to unexpected places. I could recite pages of the Dungeon Master's Handbook but was no threat on the soccer field. Even the Nerds were unwilling to accept me as one of their own. Despite an affinity for some of their practices, I simply wasn't smart enough.

I wanted to be in a gang.

Unlike our modern interpretations of thug life today, an early 80's gang concept for a poor white kid was sort of like a diluted version of the Warriors... basically a social club for bullies and losers that the rest of the world chose to ignore.

Get enough socially inept 11 year-old snot machines together and they'll form a gang. Sure, a pretend gang, with no fighting, no weapons, and not a real bully in the bunch (in fact quite the opposite), but we had a cool name, we'd draw cool slogans, and we'd have meetings. Ya know... GANG meetings, not just playing with friends, but the serious, mature stuff of talking about what teachers we didn't like and what girls we did. Finally... a purpose.

Point being, we all need tribes, and we have a lifetime to learn, or create, our roles in whatever Tribes we participate in.

So...What is a Tribe?

The concept of a tribe has an intimate appeal to it, although defining the attraction has often confounded my shallow noggin. The struggle then became to define what personal empowerment means within a tribe. How does this overtly self-centered act of physical improvement make the planet a better place? In other words, how do we save the world through deadlifts, tire flips, and tree climbing?

Of course this inquiry means defining 'tribe' beyond our camp at Burning Man or learning how to hunt a lion with spears.

According to Wikipedia, the source of all information that kinda sorta might be true, "the term is often loosely used to refer to any non-Western or indigenous society." Many anthropologists use the term to refer to societies organized largely on the basis of kinship, especially corporate descent groups. But...

> "In common modern understanding the word tribe means a social division within a traditional society consisting of a group of interlinked families or communities sharing a common culture and dialect."

Or, as Seth Godin, who literally wrote the book on tribe[15], puts it:

> *"A tribe is a group of people connected to one another, connected to a leader, and connected to an idea. For millions of years, human beings have been part of one tribe or another. A group needs only two things to be a tribe: a shared interest and a way to communicate."*

Therefore your Breakfast Club stereotypes of high school life fit the modern criteria, as would separatist groups, cults and political parties (am I being redundant?). Meanwhile the spear-hunting pagan archetype fits the more traditional view.

My romanticized version of the modern Tribe is an idealized community or society that recognizes and perpetuates 3 major tenets: Communication, Equality, and Sustainability.

Sadly these three goals are underrepresented during our current leadership (no matter who is holding what office at this moment). Communication, despite the overwhelming technology at our fingertips, seems to be dominated by the folks with the poorest forum and dialog abilities dominating what we read and hear. In other words, the dumbest are the loudest. Stupid now has volume and means. Dialectic has turned into text messaging and internet name calling and flame wars. We seem to all talk more than ever, thanks to marvelous innovations in ubiquity, yet any sort of quality filter seems to have de-evolved from our personal software. As Justin Sullivan will tell ya, *well, this Golden Age of communication means that everyone talks at the same time.*[16]

James Taylor had an interesting observation: *"The*

---

[15] Tribes: We Need You To Lead Us. Yes, you should read it.

[16] 221, by New Model Army, off of their album Thunder and Consolation. Buy it. Seriously.

information technological revolution has robbed us of the ability of making long thoughts."

Noam Chomsky considers our growing habit of shortening our information as the new censorship. We process and share the same bits on repeat, perpetuating what we already perceive without the benefit of new thought. This self inflicted newspeak isn't communication, and it builds a narrow, and delicate, peer group, one that has no longevity as an actual tribe.

This rant seems ironic after just proposing the other tenet of equality, but, let's face it, people aren't equal, as we can understand through racism and sexism. Hold on... not through actual differences in the races or genders, but because such insipid beliefs exist. Only an idiot would believe race or gender should, by right, create a hierarchy. Thus perpetrators of this myth are lacking a proper education (my polite way of saying they're morons). In a just and intellectually equal society, such tendencies to hate a fellow person for such shallow reasons would be much harder to embrace, since any rational human being with two brain cells to rub together could logically see that neither gender nor race, in themselves, have anything to do with the quality of a human being.

In our current condition, where, even awash in supposed 'communication,' it is still too easy to live in a bubble of dumb, being only influenced by like-minded chowder heads (often starting with family). The solution is education, maybe in the form of strict unconditional, judgment-free love, to eradicate deep-seated hatred based in ignorance. Have I the time, patience, or Buddha–mind for that? Lemme get back to you.

What IS equality? Let's lay the building blocks down by coveting the ability to not pass judgment on any individual due to race or gender. To keep it simple, and create a definition by what something is instead of what it isn't, could we build a tiered hierarchy of equality, not unlike Maslow's hierarchy of needs?

Tier one could be an open acceptance of gender and race.
Tier 2: acceptance of religion or system of belief (this includes sexuality).
Tier 3: acceptance of behavior and decisions
Tier 4: turning acceptance into respect, appreciation, and dialog, often referred to as understanding.

What is this acceptance stuff we're harping on about here? Well we've discussed physical foundations, but for our purpose to reek of hylomorphism, we've gotta carve in stone some metaphysical foundations to strive for.

The big three recommended here would be Accepting, Sharing, and Becoming.

Let's get a few things understood about acceptance. It isn't a passive state. It is truly a verb, just like you are. It seems contrary to accept what we don't agree with. It battles our social mores to accept a structure or belief that is contrary to ours, in someone else, or sometimes even ourselves (remember that cognitive dissonance we chatted about earlier?).

Acceptance isn't conformity. It isn't kowtowing to something as a subservient marshmallow. It is simply an understanding of the present moment free from the filters of emotion, hope, or that nasty cognitive dissonance. It is a highly active observation, not a reactive judgment. Only then can we begin to assess, adapt, adjust, adopt, or avoid. Only then can we transform.

Acceptance isn't romanticizing or celebrating a scenario either. That seems to be a popular reaction to shame. A behavior with serious risks involved often becomes a glorified identity, shared on social media with volume and pride.

Instead, accept, than transform. Accepting and then glorifying can be antithetical to usefulness.

We can't transform what we don't believe exists. Know your Now, then make the changes needed. Accepting isn't synonymous with 'being OK with it." Knowing the difference is important. Accepting is acknowledging what is, sans judgment. Acceptance is understanding the truth for that moment. Then you can transform as will benefit you and your tribe.

Acceptance has one profound action that will bridge all three driving parts of the hylomorphic self. Many folks smarter than I would make a case that acceptance often begins with a big dollop of forgiveness. As mentioned, we might define strength as love. Forgiveness is also high on the list of things we can define strength as.

Sharing

So throughout this book I've quoted Tommy Kono[17]. Let's chat more about him.

To generations preceding my own, Tommy Kono is often remembered with profound reverence. His history is easy to research, but in summary: championship weightlifter and bodybuilder through the late 50s. My gym, BodyTribe Fitness, isn't far from the home in which a young Tommy trained for the Olympics in a basement with a dusty floor and low ceilings, so there's an almost tactile geography that connects us. I'm from Hawaii and now live in Sacramento. He was the opposite. We lived quite close to where the other grew up, even if there is about 40 years that separates us chronologically. But as much as his history intrigues me, the opportunity to extend his legacy is an opportunity I hold dearer. I'll never be even close to the caliber of lifter Tommy was. Heck, very few will ever reach 3 Olympic medals, 6 world championships, and a dozen or so world records. No, the legacy I have is the honor of carrying on

---

[17] Tommy Kono left us on April 24th, 2016, right after I wrote this passage. My heart was heavy when I went through the edit and changed the tenses from current to past. He was an important part of BodyTribe and is deeply missed.

is his three simple words, which, by now, will look familiar to anyone reading this book.

Practice makes permanent.

All of the lifting cues, all of the technique tweaks, all of the mental game he'd taught me over the years were simply extensions of this one law. In my perpetual quest to embody a bridge between mind, body, and spirit, this lesson now permeates every aspect of my journey. Any result we ever get is the culmination of this law, whether we like it or not, whether we believe it or not.

From the workshops I teach across the country, to the friends and clients within my local network, this idea of the permanence of what we practice is repeated, and drilled, in any lesson I impart, preserving the legacy of Tommy Kono in every student I encounter. From Tommy, I've learned that the information is what is important, more so than the teacher. He wanted the ideas, the techniques, the philosophy of strength to inspire people, not a name, a face, or a celebrity status.

An important point to know about Tommy, which transcends his well documented lifting history: he never asked for a dime for any of the time he spent teaching us. He never left empty handed, since I made sure everyone handed over $20 for the honor of literally sitting at the feet of the master, which meant I was able to make the trip have some financial value for him. But, from day one, the money wasn't the issue. For Tommy, the knowledge needed sharing. And, even well into his 80s, he sat and chatted with us, sometimes a group of 30+ eager minds and bodies, for several hours, often even coaching us hands-on through some lifting. Tommy's practice was giving.

Which is a lesson in itself, especially for a journey of strength and movement. Practice isn't always physical. It isn't always even easily tangible. Sometimes it's just being good to each other.

22. Sustainability

In San Francisco, the city where Tony Bennett left his heart, an annual event takes place that allows mere mortals like myself to listen to, and get the required social media documentation of, Dr. Jane Goodall, DBE, the Mary Wollstonecraft of animal rights. Being that our little movement sanctuary, BodyTribe, is a pretty big player on the local animal rescue circuit, several of us tend to make the trek to see her, and to become sponges of compassion for Dr. Goodall's words to work their magic.

One of my partners in crime at BodyTribe is head trainer Allyson Seconds, a noted animal activist in her own right. She studies Dr. Goodall with a fangirl passion that is more recognizable in sci-fi geeks having a profound relationship with every plot line of Firefly. In her healthy obsession (no cosplay costume... yet), she noticed a basic model that Dr. Goodall followed that was bold in its simplicity and revolutionary in the possibilities to turn our mess around a bit. Al pointed out that Jane focused on the three basics, which, much to my dismay were NOT the aforementioned BodyTribe staples of Train Well, Eat Well, and Rest Well.

They were indeed:

Animals.

Humans.

Nature.

Them's the big three. As mentioned earlier, one of them is not crucial to the survival of the other two, despite the fact that it's the one that has grandiose views of being the leader of a hierarchy with the other two ranking considerably lower in the pecking order. Ironically, the other two are quite crucial to the extended dance party of the arrogant one.

Perhaps our extra RAM and amazing DSL connection between body and mind were installed to keep our comparatively weak and ugly flesh packets on an even playing ground. Therefore our technological advancements lack merit in the big picture when they become tools of total domination over the other two groups. With only a modicum of investigation we could probably link many of our major health issues (and a handful of political issues) to throwing our causal relationship into disarray in our quest for total control. Jeez, give us an inch, and we'll try to take over the universe.

Allyson's theory on our role transcends inward from the big picture down to the individual person when we start tying the actual ability of our bodies into the equation. Each body, each physical flesh packet, is in itself an ecosystem. Once we grok this, the big picture might make more sense, as would the role of movement and strength, and competition as empowerment, in supporting not just our personal planet, but the actual big earthy one we all hang out on.

Makes me wanna gnaw on these words of Al's:

There is no perfection, just purity.

If we can't be proper caretakers of our personal ecosystem, how can we expect our roles in the tribal ecosystem, and then the planetary ecosystems, to even matter? Are we useful? To ourselves, others, and the planet?

Sustainability means not destroying our planet. Easy, right? If authentic strength is the relationship between ourselves and our bodies, and eventually ourselves and the tribe, then fitness is not only the sustainability of our personal ecosystems, but a step towards tribal sustainability as well.

As the epicenter of a small concept in movement philosophy, I'm now trying to see my/our place within the tribe.

How can I add to those three tenets through the rituals of my sanctuary?

This big picture dreaming is what I relegate as homework for all the attendees of our strength camps and workshops. Fitness is currently sold as an individual, ego-based pursuit. Get buff = get laid/get recognized/get money/get stuff. That message doesn't address how the tribe benefits? How can society increase its capability through our individual fitness endeavors?

Remember the technique for defining strength and fitness? That's how you can begin to answer that question.

With this in mind, the tribe can only exist if unified in compassion and support. The components of fitness as defined by the physical subculture - strength, courage, persistence, etc. - can only succeed if they come from a foundation of sharing. How a tribe differs from modern clans, clubs, or parties is that the support and compassion needs to be inclusive, extending to anyone, not just tribal members.

Remember, a healthy tribe, even if it doesn't have much, shares as naturally as we breathe.

As mentioned, when I teach a workshop or meet with a new client, their first task is to define the words 'strength' and 'fitness,' and define it for themselves, making their concept of it unique and personal. This inspection starts them on their individual, and perpetual, quest for their own movement philosophy. Yeah, I know, sounds totally exciting, doesn't it?

Well, we think it's cool. But then what? Personal empowerment can't exist in a vacuum, unless, of course, living alone in a Hoover is your personal kink. Maslow's hierarchy pyramid, which should be shaped differently to represent 'actualization' as a big open door into the universe, is sometimes modified to include self-transcendence beyond (above) self-actualization. Some describe this as an egoless wisdom, where the intense emotional roadblocks associated with lack of movement from the lower parts of the hierarchy no longer exist.

In other words, the cool kids are soooo above anger, jealousy, and fear. Only losers still dwell in these reactive impulses. Heck, maybe at that point it would be obvious as to how such empowerment relates to the tribe, but I'm not going to assume too many answers at this point. If Maslow's hierarchy was a flight of stairs, I'm buying new hiking boots and an extra large Camelbak for the remaining trek I have.

If we can fathom a tribe being a society larger than the 4 friends with personalized ring tones in your phone, then a general truth I'm starting to absorb now is that being a badass without the tribe in mind is NOT being a badass.

Hey, geographically our modern networks can be spread all over the place, which defies the traditional sense of a tribe in terms of proximity. Support still openly exists, if we actually use the modern communication technologies for tribal sustainability. How can we meet the three tenets of a thriving tribe? That's the underlying premise of this book. Everything seems to come back to...

Body: Foundations and explorations of movement and strength
Community: Protect, Provide, Play
Culture: Accept, Share, Become

23. The Full Circle

"Knowing is not enough. We must apply." - Johann Wolfgang von Goethe

I blame powerlifter Dave Tate for putting the original germ of this idea in my noggin, which has since been washed around by the spam and lime jello between my ears into my "concept of perpetual learning," or, to borrow from my guru terminology kit, the "Principle of Continuing Education."

The Full Circle is the alchemic formula that transforms learning into knowing, and knowing into Becoming. We stockpile an impressive menagerie of learning daily. Often we're one step away from being information hoarders, stuffing our skulls with enough data flotsam that our brains have a tough time finding the remote to our inner eye's big screen. In other words we learn stuff all the time, but that is only part of the journey around the full circle. Learning is not knowing, just like having a gym membership, gym shoes, gym shorts, and a gym bag is not actually working out. Learning is simply the acquiring of information.

Take a look at your own personal biography. Think back to 4th grade, for example. There was a heap o' lurnin' to be done, but I'll bet my used undies you don't know everything you learned back then. In my case I don't remember how to properly diagram a sentence (as might be horribly evident), but

I could tell you all about a brontosaurus[18]. Why? I came Full Circle with dinosaurs, but English composition took a priority just above having rocks thrown at me and a bit below wondering what these fascinating creatures called girls were all about.

The Full Circle starts with, of course, the desire to know something. If that curiosity isn't there, education halts, since a lack of enthusiasm for the knowledge means an aborted quest, even if the information if freely abundant. When our passion to nerd-up on something does kick in, when we crave the knowing, we must begin by learning. Then we make the climb up one side of the circle, where we read, listen, and fill our heads with the desired information.

But then? Oh, but then!! Then we come back down the other side, putting this fresh, newly acquired data in action. We Apply!

In the gym, the Full Circle might begin by memorizing every article on whatever the current click-bait version of T-Nation happens to be, collecting certifications, or even spending years earning your degree. But all of it doesn't means squat... literally, since nothing in your brain will prepare you to squat until you actually SQUAT. We need Time Under The Bar, as it is known by coaches world wide (Under The Bar is even the name of Dave Tate's tome of powerlifting motivation), or The TUB Principle, as we'll call it. This is where learning becomes knowledge, where a true iron head understands that all the schooling they've been feeding their brains has no place except as reference material for the real action of actual force development. (Yes, this applies to just about anything. Swimmer? Time in the Water. Climber? Time on the Mountain.)

---

[18] Now known as the Apatosaurus, for the astute and pedantic amongst you... yeah, and Pluto's not a planet? C'mon!

Then 'twould behoove us to have in place a system of awareness that then applies our knowledge to life, completing the circle with holomorphic understanding of the information.

We learn it, apply it to our training and then apply it to life. That's the full circle, and we have to start at the beginning of the circle every time we embark on learning/knowing/becoming something new, in the gym or out in that scary world beyond the iron.

How did this work with the brontosaurus in the 5th grade? Books and films were fun and all, but getting covered in sand and mud with my models and toys of the giant lizards was my true research, and made more effective by everything I read. I *was* a dinosaur (some say I still am), and I wanted nostrils on the top of my head too. I *knew* about dinosaurs. And I *became* an active, playful, curious human being.

Take a few trips around the Full Circle, and you'll hone a discerning mind, making the trip up the first half of the circle quicker. You'll assimilate information efficiently, testing it against what your noggin and body already know, letting superfluous information fall aside while having a well-tuned application process that can put the absconded information into personal law much faster than anything our government has ever achieved.

Learn, apply, become, learn, apply, become, over and over, for the rest of our lives.

If enough people made the journey around this circle, the fitness trend industry would crumble. The Full Circle creates a level of wisdom that separates those who've made the journey enough times to know better from those who follow a program without questioning it, or still post on internet fitness forums looking for exercises to 'tone the lower abs.'

The Full Circle of Training will always bring us back to the three basics:

Train Well
Eat Well
Rest Well

How DO I train well, eat well and rest well? Now the answers aren't as easy, because any answer is useless unless processed through the Full Circle. To the dismay of many, that takes work.

Become

> More than "attacking fat" and "blasting muscles" training is about appreciating the simple wonder of being. All the angry, punishing vitriol around fitness is egoic projection of a crippled domination mindset wrapped in self-loathing and fear. Loving compassion for oneself will bring greater results than an antagonistic hammering.
> -Steven Blondeau

We are more verb than noun. More action than object. Around the circle we go.

24. Tribes and Traditions

Filiopietistic. An archaic enough word that my spell check doesn't even recognize it. It's the great, and possibly *too* great, reverence for tradition. Our government recently decided that any two individuals may marry each other. The groundbreaking part of this decision was the battle won against the *filiopietistic* idea that those two people had to be of opposite genders. As a country we kicked gravity's ass with such force that our feet touched the moon 47 years ago, but we were still mired in a stale tradition that may once have had practical roots a kajillion years ago. The classic blueprint seemed to be: Grab the nearest person of the opposite gender, shack up, get freaky, and grow your tribe by making more copies of yourself.

Making a case for this idea now is only argued by hand picked parts of religious doctrine.

Our big party bus, the modern American tribe, doesn't have to rely on dusty traditions to keep its wheels turning. Marriage, gender roles, traditional hierarchies... none serve the role of cultural durability that made them so supposedly gosh darn crucial the centuries before us. Choosing to hold onto them is simply that... a choice. They are no longer a requirement for perceived tribal survival, despite how badly you want to believe otherwise.

For every pundit of the good ol' days rallying around the

flag of 'traditional values', there is someone who, although not always entirely conscious of their path, is stepping away from previous societal habits and dancing a different jig, since the bounty and growth of the tribe is no longer dependent on the original, time-honored-but-kinda-boring (or outright wrong) steps.

Out of this grows the fungus of smaller, more intimate tribes, folks who agree on new standards for the fuel of their new, improved party bus.

Oh, some of the classics are still crucial... be nice to each other, fill bellies who are hungry, have fair and just dialog... symptoms of the successful tribal existence (which I've blabbed about a bit ago): sustainability, communication, and equality. When a tradition exists that is superfluous to the evolution of the tribe, though, holding on to it (or not) is, or at least should be, an individual decision.

Worse, though, is the tradition that actually contradicts current societal empowerment. Our current political/cultural structure is rife with this unjustified cultural baggage, no matter what side you're standing on. That little diatribe will be for a different day. I'm putting my soapbox away after one more little observation.

Strength doesn't slip into the role of gratuitous tradition! It is still essential. There has yet to be made a good case for being weak. I'm guessing there won't be any time soon.

Modern Traditions: What is the Physical SubCulture?

As will be repeated throughout this little pastiche, we can't achieve, teach or seek what isn't defined, except through beautiful incidents of accidental Zen. Although often fluky, no book or idea of mine shall ever bear the yoke of being 'beautiful.' Or Zen.

The term 'physical subculture' was first used as the title of an article written about my gym, BodyTribe Fitness. Jimmy Calanchini, a mohawked journalist/musician, coined the term after spending some time listening to my endless patter about the need to return to the roots of fitness, the physical culture movement of a century or so ago.

Jimmy shared some of my biases against the current corporate fitness structure, and with both of us having a bit of a punk rock past, our dialog soon met on common ground about the need for a grassroots movement for change. The physical culture has been relegated to an underground movement, what health coach Cody Fielding and I joke about as the 'Movement movement,' and Jimmy termed the Physical Subculture.

Physical culture was what the fitness movement was before it became a product. Originally, the Physical Culture was empowerment through movement, not the attempt of superficial pride through mirrors and scales. You looked strong, powerful, or 'in shape' because you *were*, a concept based on passion for ability, now lost in the vacant sea of skin-deep obligations, eating disorders, and Orwellian joy drugs.

The body is a tool for greater purpose, not just the end result of your training. Therefore, training is the means to increase the quality of life through movement, which is how I define the word "Fitness." The Physical SubCulture movement is the modern organized effort to incorporate centuries of physical rituals and beliefs in exercise and movement into an integral part of all aspects of culture. Whether through lifting heavy objects of all shapes and sizes or finding new ways to move the body by itself, the Physical SubCulture movement is about strengthening the spirit through pushing the limits of the body, therefore creating useful members of your tribe.

Why a subculture? Simple. We're independent from the mainstream modern fitness industry, practicing and playing almost as an underground movement against the modern corporate structure. About a century ago, the quest for strength and ability WAS the fitness movement, and Physical Culture was the banner it fell under.

What went wrong? Since more money can be made from

trying to sell the quest for aesthetic perfection and exploiting exercise as the snake oil for 'beauty,' a distorted, and limited, view of exercise and training has emerged: the obligatory path to a better appearance, or, to be blunt, a gym membership is simply part of the war chest in the quest to get laid. As we mentioned before, if sex sells, then increasing the possibility of sex sells even more. Earlier we were crass enough to call it fuckability.

Marketing and promoting of exercise as the magical tool for achieving ultimate sexy status helped usher in decades of self-image woes and issues that have created entire industries to both feed and cure low self esteem (and give therapists job security for centuries). The formula was easy, and is still used today (look at any 'health and fitness' magazine cover). Remember the equation that has proven an effective moneymaker for commercial gyms and supplement companies for many years? We mentioned this one a couple times already:

"You are ugly. We can help."

This marketing formula sure works better in our society than trying to sell the Physical Culture concept of movement; that physical strength and performance increase other qualities of life as well. Looking good, which apparently comes in a bottle or within 3 easy payments for some infomercial gadget that can give you instant results just by looking at it collect dust in your bedroom, is an easier sell than *being* good, which, aside from being a great deal of work, is free.

As Bernarr MacFadden used as a slogan for his Physical Culture magazine that he started in 1899, "Weakness is a Crime – Don't be a Criminal."

Movement should be that integral to our existence, but not through the obligation of aesthetics. Over time the performance and ability of the body, which has a direct and strong impact on the spirit and mind, took a minor role in training. Today, the commercial 'fitness' industry is a sham, selling the distractions of gadgets, supplements, and imagery, not actual exercise or ability. The mere fact that such things as 'ab' machines exist just proves how silly the industry has become. Even the alt-fitness world, that nouveau trend of what looks like real work with real tools in industrial spaces, still promotes and perpetuates aesthetic stereotypes while providing little in embodiment.

The Physical Culture movement has always been around, though. It just may be hard to find these days. It has become a subculture, a movement forcing the mainstream to evaluate what training really is.

What is the Physical Subculture? This is not a complete list...

- A passion for strength, not an obligation of the scale.
- Training without mirrors, without fads, without judgment.
- Understanding the mind and spirit better through movement.
- Often picking up something heavy. Really heavy.
- No fear of the body's abilities.
- Using REAL training tools with long histories. No gadgets or trends.
- Embracing training as playtime. Life changing playtime.
- Acknowledging and exploring capability.
- Training techniques that are useful, enjoyable, and sacred.
- Banishing weakness.

25. How to Become Ambassadors for Change?

Anyone
Someone
Everyone
I dreamt this. According to this dream, these were the same words found on a napkin given to the guitar player of a classic punk band by their singer the night they both died. At least that's what it said in my dead rock star guide book that I was using as a connect-the-dots map while I toured around LA. And yes, I dream in color.

But I digress. It was quite a dream.

"Chip" is not on my birth certificate. It was bestowed upon me at birth, though, and although it lacks the respectability of being on that important document, I do consider it my 'real' name (mostly through familiarity, not by winning any cool points). This title juggling is not my exclusive party; a great percentage of my friends refer to themselves with names other than the moniker that claims first chair on their early paperwork.

Imagine, if you will, being in a position of such great respect (or in a mind-numbing ego trip) that you would answer to the name Guru of the Blissful Refuge. There are two important things you should do to earn such a name, and if you guessed becoming a guru, and having a pretty groovy pad, so groovy in fact, that you could label it not only a refuge, but a blissful one at that, then you're correct.

Recently some words from someone who actually does answer to that very name for reals jumped into my consciousness and held a forum there. The good Swami, a devotee of Bhakti yoga, was a highlighted subject of a recent documentary on modern yoga practices, called Enlighten Up. The film's premise was to take a neophyte to yoga and steep him in it with the goal of discovering enlightenment. The filmmaker and director, herself a long time practitioner of yoga, hadn't apparently tapped into this cosmic happiness yet. Due to her failure at achieving whatever 'it' is, she'd try to see what she was missing by getting a newbie to find 'it.'

Although beautifully filmed, the movie fell tragically short of its intended premise. Or did it? The fascinating final interview with the aforementioned Guru so blatantly laid out the differences of western thought and the original concepts of yoga, it was a little shocking when the film's subject, and the film's director, missed the point entirely.

Enlightenment, like fitness, wealth, heck, success in general, is a very individual pursuit in our culture, often using fancy language like "actualization" to veil a selfishness in the quest. We *seek* enlightenment; we search for it; we build personal campaigns to *find* it (and make documentaries of the process). It is a path to *rise above*. A concept that seems to be a very Western goal, this rising above. We find all sorts of ways to attempt it, and we have strong judgments on the value of the goal. To rise above at the cost of others suffering, through greed, domination, or violence is bad. On the other hand, rising above through this supposedly benign pursuit of enlightenment would wear a more positive badge. We'd call it 'good.'

To the bhakta, one who follows the *bhakti marga* – the bhakti way – 'enlightenment' has nothing to do with searching, finding, or rising above. In fact the root of yoga, the actual meaning of the word, is to 'come together;' in their case, to come together with God. Do not make the mistake that God is referred to as a literal higher being, one that coming together with would mean 'rising above' the riffraff of humanity. The idea is much less exclusively divine, and way more bonding than that. The many bhakta referenced in the movie never once called God 'him' or 'it,' but rather 'everything.' God as the ultimate Tribe, free of many of our western religious ideologies. We don't 'rise above' to understand our relation to this tribe, this planet, this universe... we simply 'come together' with it.

John Lennon was onto something.

How did the Guru answer the redundant questions of 'what do I do and how do I do it?' He repeated:

Be you.

What does this mean?

"As much as possible, try to get rid of what you are not."

The basic BodyTribe Premise is to ask WHY. Everyone in the fitness industry will give you their version of How and What, but where are the folks asking WHY?! We need to. Thankfully, the Guru of the Blissful Refuge agrees...

> *"It's not important what you are doing. It's important WHY you are doing. You can prepare food for just consuming. You can prepare food for someone you love. And you can prepare food for your Ishta, your Bhagwan... the Lord. So the action will be the same, Physically. But inside it is different. If you are forced to do some cooking for someone you don't like, then you will do it... you will cook. But you won't enjoy it."*

Yup.

> *"You came to meet me. You could have come by cycle, you could have come by car, you could have come by elephant, you could have come by foot. To reach here,*

*there are so many directions. That depends on you,
where you are present. Because... you are the most, or
let me use my word, most-est, important person under
the sun."*

Or, as Lennon wrote...

*Dear Prudence, open up your eyes
Dear Prudence, see the sunny skies
The wind is low, the birds will sing
That you are part of everything
Dear Prudence, won't you open up your eyes?
Look around*

Anyone
Someone
Everyone

My mystic dream napkin made perfect sense:

You are not Anyone, you are Someone. As Someone, you
are not just Anyone, You are Everyone.

Be the ambassador of movement to your tribe simply by
striving to be the best you, or the *most* you possible. Being you
should be what you're best at, yet we distract ourselves from
this potent ability, consciously and less-than-consciously. Our
training, as a vehicle for mindfulness, as an expression of our
curiosity, and as an exploration of possibility, will then be an
example of how the hylomorphic self becomes an important,
dare I say *useful*, member of any tribe we're part of.

Am I useful? I dunno, but I'm working on it.

26. The Importance of #2

(Intensity through Purpose)

If you've made it this far, then you have a tenacity of spirit that gives you bragging rights. Despite conceit not being a particularly embodied trait, sometimes we can all use a little strut. You've actually declared, whether you know it or not, that you have a true passion for movement and strength. Training is not just a hobby. You're now waist-deep in your pursuit of Why, which is the perfect time to change the question.

How does training work? You know... metaphysically?

Training, when taken to its holistic conclusion, is an awareness of the self and our relationship to the tribe. This embodiment is, of course, what any deep passion has the power to become. What's unique about our movement and strength practice is that it has this profound, hylomorphic process waiting to be exposed while also being a truly tactile experience. We build some good ol' useable physical skills in the process.

Again, how does this metaphysical part work? Empowerment isn't automatic. When delving into the What, you'll find a bunch of beautiful training protocols that, as physical skill building templates, are the real deal. But without the goal of Becoming, without the presence to embody that goal, they won't ultimately be transformative. The folks who succeed do so because of something that is beyond the physical. Frankly, almost any program can offer some degree of insight into the self if we're ready to embrace what I call Step #2. We're just often too quick to buy into the distraction, the false awareness. We lose our way, and pay good money to do so.

Step One: Steal underpants.

Remember this South Park episode? When asked why the underpants gnomes were stealing and hoarding the kid's underpants, said gnomes produced a chart.

Step 1) Steal underpants
Step 2)
Step 3) Profit!

This basic template, just with different wording, is an accurate representation of how we believe automatic success works, and we buy it in many forms. Now 'automatic' doesn't mean instantaneous. No, we have to work for the 'profit.' But we believe this hard work *automatically* begets something successful, something desired. The fitness industrial complex sells it to us this way...

Step 1) Workout
Step 2)
Step 3) A better you!

Without a defined Step #2 your outcome may as well be based on dreams and rainbow rides. Snorting all the pixie dust you can squeeze out of hippy poop will give you as much chance of success as not having a plan. The Fitness Industrial Complex has no Step 2. What's your Step 2?

As we've rambled on about, we'd better define a purpose. Maybe this doesn't have to happen before Step 1, but somewhere pretty close on the timeline. A good goal would be to make purpose an integral part of Step 1.

Step 2 is simple, yet endlessly complex: Be Aware. This skill, however, as any neuroscientist or meditation mentor could tell you, is no easy task.

The wordy version:

Step 1) Workout (with purpose)

Step 2) Create awareness of self, perpetuating a greater understanding, respect, and appreciation of our relationship with my body.

Step 3) A better Me!

Yeah, that's a mouthful. Let's boil Step 2 down into three sections To paraphrase some words of wisdom, you can spend the rest of your life trying to understand just one of these, and it would not be a life wasted.

Step 2:

- Be present.
- Turn judgment into observation.
- Find joy/appreciation.

Be present.

When everything is a race, we forget that the view might be beautiful.

I begin my workshops with a simple, yet deeply profound (in my mind) little movement drill that begins the relationship with awareness.

We roll. We grab our knees (our own... that should be clarified), and we roll, in any and every direction we can. Once we're all oddly shaped balls, the game of exploration begins. Our adult recess opens up a series of relationships, first between this group and myself. It's my way of reading the room. An assessment that stands on its own of how the group will synchronize, and of how the individuals will respond to an important question, a question that identifies the next relationship: the individuals with themselves.

It's a question I'll ask again and again: "Any Observations?"

Another important relationship we can assess from this seemingly goofy drill is the relationship of the group as, well, a group. Beyond my relationship with them, this bit of exploration recess will result in a quick summary of how they work as a unit. Are they playful? Is there laughter? Is there contact (or the avoidance of it)?

My So-Called Virtual Life

Situational awareness is a term that might be described by the bookish as a *pleonasm*, which is a fun word not just because it should be in a hip hop song rhymed with *orgasm*. Situational awareness usually refers to a preparedness related to danger and potential combat, but that leaves us with no separate term to describe the art of being prepared for beauty, adventure, compassion, or, simply, anything else. Since all relationships - personal, interpersonal, and with space and time - change according to environment or circumstance, i.e. via the situation, the case can be made that awareness is always situational, and all situations require awareness, therefore making the category of situational awareness... well, pleonastic.[19]

Awareness by any name is a dying art, since our virtual world is destroying all of it. The illiterates of the next century are those who cannot participate in real life. They can read words, but their reading comprehension of life will straight up suck.

Thinking is the awareness of the brain, not the body. Sometimes thinking has to step to the side. Which brings us to a tough fact to accept.

---

[19] The song would be called *Pleonasty*, by the way. Yes, it would be amazing.

When it comes to movement, your brain can be a bit of a moron. Your body is the genius. It learns movement faster than your thought process lets it. Our adult brains over-think intense movement in the same way we complicate all of our relationships. To thwart, or at least reduce, this reaction, the authentic performance model, where our body is most productive, is centered on a surprisingly tricky concept when it comes to training:

Turning Judgment into observation.

Letting the somatic nervous system do its thing without negative interference from the autonomic nervous systems. Or, in simple terms, not letting the brain's prejudices interfere with the body's practices. How about an example from the iron?

Strength sports, which, for the uninitiated, would be the classification of competitions where people hoist, throw, carry, or flip really heavy things[20] is rife with crucial moments where observation and judgment collide. In playing with a heavy barbell, for instance, the first pull of a snatch[21] is a defining moment of your movement meditation skills.

Getting the bar from the ground to the thigh is a comparatively slow part of the entire complex of the snatch, but still takes less than a second even for many slower, newer lifters. Within that brief time frame your mad young Jedi skills can make or break the lift, depending on whether the weight being moved is *judged* as heavy, or simply *observed* as heavy.

As a judgment, our amazing brains will then quantify the

---

[20] If you guessed powerlifting or strongman, for instance, you may not be a complete neophyte to this brand of battle. If you immediately thought of golf, though, your understanding of both 'strength' and 'sport' is now being seriously called into question.

[21] If you are unfamiliar with the snatch, please make sure to add the words 'olympic lift' into the Google search or you will be setting yourself up distraction. Possibly hours of it.

weight as something potentially bad or undesirable. Now here's the thing... if the brain speaks up (say, like a judgment), the body listens and reacts. If the brain judges the lift 'heavy,' then the body understands that to mean challenging, and not in the good way. As a judgment, heavy = this sucks. The body reacts accordingly, by either anticipating the dangerous, heavy weight by tightening up for it (and screwing up the lift, the lifting equivalent of a flinch), or simply giving up too soon.

'Heavy' as an observation, though, has no negative impact on the body. The body simply doesn't care, since no quality has been defined, and therefore the brain has introduced no emotion from prejudice. If the brain just steps out of the way and observes 'heavy,' the body has no obstacle beyond practiced talent.

The skill of non-judgment is what often separates veteran competitors from newbies. The battle-scared lifter can just observe the fact that it is heavy. *Of course* it's heavy. That's why we're here. So the brain can simply watch from afar and let the body do what it's supposed to. Butch Curry[22] calls it *lifting stupid*. The understanding that the brain, after being part of the initial skill learning, now doesn't know best and better get out of the way when it's time to actually perform the skill.

A metaphor for life? You make the call. Do we need to get the heck out of our heads sometimes and just live? Passion demands it.

Adults stink at this. Children have a much more wonderfully naïve concept of judgment when it comes to movement, not letting it hinder their exploration. We adulticize movement, letting our grown up brains boss our bodies around, getting in the way of actually learning and growing through a profound, yet erroneous level of rationalization or judgment. In the rolling game that begins my workshops, we're quick to observe how challenging this simple

[22] Former Olympic team member and current iron guru.

movement request is. On paper our tumbling is a rather childish drill. But the amount of brain that steps in to try to direct the action creates more problems than solutions. The body, which is playful and experimental by nature (child-like), grumbles and struggles against the judgments and obstacles created by the brain. That's adultisizing, and it often ruins not just performance, but fun[23].

Getting to know ourselves a bit better will have to involve less talk, more rock, so to speak. Involve the body in the discussion, and sit the brain down and tell it to shut up and listen.

Living Longer versus Dying Longer

Sometimes our lives are blessed with heroes, like the folks who conquer life-threatening illnesses with dignity and wisdom. Disease survivors offer insight into perseverance and compassion that any tribe can benefit from.

Then there's the bigger population of *diseased* survivors, the culture busy barely surviving life. Modern medicine can keep them alive despite their journeys full of choices to the contrary. We're the healthiest sick people ever. We're not living longer. We're dying longer. Our periods of disconnect with our bodies are simply elongated.

Climb, play, love, dance, swim, mate, fly... connect with yourself (heck, maybe even with someone else) today. Chat with your body a bit. Live longer rather than die longer.

Where do the greatest joys of training come from? Meeting the brain's obligations or the body's desires?

Step 2 means train to live, not live to train.

---

[23] Adulticize is a little different from Bonnie Prudden's Adulticide, though we both laughed when we discovered we came up with similar terms to explain similar processes.

27. Thank You

(Intensity Through Inspiration)

Every time I travel to teach, my first stop in the new town is a grocery store. Besides learning a great deal about the demographic of the neighborhood I'm staying in, the local food mart has an open invitation to the old art of people watching. Consider these excursions primal social media. When you discover the right frequency for tuning into live-action humanity, you're filled with something a bit greater than just hitting a 'like' button.

Recently there was a man in front of me in the checkout line. He was a big man. Not the kind of big that comes as the enviable outcome of choices made in the gym. More like his past decisions involved many foods that were probably in plastic wrap and were of colors not entirely natural. He wore these decisions as considerable extra weight. Some of his history was now unwanted aesthetic carriage.

He became the reason I moved and celebrated movement that weekend. He was my lesson.

He was a true shining example of how training can infect our tribes as a tool of empowerment. I didn't meet him. I simply overheard and witnessed a few choice words and actions and decided that he was my mentor for that moment.

He had a son, probably 3 years old. In our short time sharing space (I was behind them for less than 4 minutes), dad made it clear that he was now creating a newer, different journey, one that was meant to include, educate, and inspire his son. His personal empowerment will now be through his role in empowering this small tribe of family. From within earshot I picked up that at least part of it had to do with training, movement, and good food choices (I peeked in his cart, as I do everyone near me in line at the grocery store. Even as I try to reserve judgment, I'm usually disappointed. Not today.).

He had a goal. It was obvious and uplifting. I'm sure superficially it had to do with fat loss and wellness boosting, but those will actually be symptoms of his journey. The actual transformation, the true success, will happen if the scale needle moves a little or a lot. Someone else is involved. Someone else will learn and improve. In his mission, at least two are loved (probably more).

Living for the gym, and using the gym to live are two incredibly different things. He personified how the physical begets the metaphysical. He was, in my definition of the word, strong.

The coveted physical changes of intense movement – strength, shape, performance – are simply adaptations to perpetuate more of it. Movement is the tactile exploration of space. It is knowing where you are, and who you are, through participation. Our body adapts to strength training by getting better at it, with the main purpose of being able to move and do more

At least that is the original purpose for our organic machines. Sure, free will dictates you can do with it as you please, but remember that better choices now mean more choices later. Why not use it for what it was intended?

For someone like my new friend in the grocery store, this new journey, these fresh decisions he now makes every day, are quite possibly as challenging and as scary as a veteran lifter attempting a new PR. Probably more so.

How is he, then, not strong?

Us versus Us

These pains that you feel are messengers.
Listen to them. Turn them to sweetness. The night
is almost over. You were young once, and content.
Now you think about money all the time.
You used to be that money. You were a healthy vine. Now
you're a rotten fruit. You ought to be growing sweeter
and sweeter, but you've gone bad.   - Rumi

To paraphrase Henry Rollins, 100 pounds doesn't change, just your relationship to it does.

You can't always change your situation, but you can change your relationship to it. You can't always change your body - yeah, you're always gonna have troll feet, yes, your ears are sorta stuck that way, no, you cannot have supermodel proportions, sorry you're always gonna be that height – but you can change your relationship with it.

How great is life when there are still surprises daily for our enjoyment and wonder. Bodytribe is a strength dojo for the folks who have to work hard for their superhero status. We've got some naturally gifted folk, to be sure; folks to inspire and motivate us kinda average, darn-my-less-than-uber-parents-for-my-struggling-genetics sort of people. Many of us, with a big finger pointed directly at my own semi-sunken chest, didn't ace the presidential fitness tests in school (hey, someone needs to form the big hump in the middle of the bell curve) and would be lumped among the statistical category at any corporate gym as simply "paying member," with no fanfare or possibility of ever making it into any of their promotional literature.

Let this be my big Thank You to my fellow 'average' folks who constantly blow me away with the effort, sweat, and maybe a little blood they donate to their humble sanctuary. Upon my exit from my dojo every day ("Thank you for keeping me humble and strong" I say as I bow) I have a new batch of memories of greatly satisfying accomplishments of our tribe. New skills being honed to take home to your other tribes, gained through great effort and great satisfaction. I find ongoing inspiration in your successes.

The constant quest for inspiration and motivation beyond yourself often blinds you to yourself. Inside you is a cosmic nuclear reactor: fission, fusion, and frantic power. Take it. Use it. Trust it. It's not out there in the books you read or the quotes you post. It's the universal goo that pumps from your heart. It's the vibrating potential energy hiding in your muscles. It's the inertia in the bones and the fire in the most sophisticated communication system available... your central nervous system.

You are the sweet chant of frantic power. Let's hear it.

It's more Why than What. Sure, it's your body. Move it. Move the shit out of that body. But know why, or stop wasting your time.

About the Author:

In this book you've been privy to my love of animals, my strength athletic journeys, my childishness, and even some personal history about swimming, love, and roll playing games. How much more do you want? You may have garnered that I run a gym in Sacramento called BodyTribe Fitness. Perhaps you gleaned that I have a musical background. Currently I teach, write, create videos, and spend time with my girlfriend, 3 dogs, and a cat. I'm Facebook-friendly and might even have a twitter account.

I make a fine vegan mac-n-cheese but still can't quite nail down the secret of a good malai kofta.

Made in the USA
Middletown, DE
08 March 2020